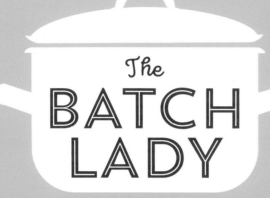

HEALTHY FAMILY FAVOURITES

TO EVERYONE WHO STRUGGLES DAILY WITH HAVING TO GET
A MEAL ON THE TABLE, AND IS FOREVER ANSWERING THE
QUESTION, 'WHAT'S FOR DINNER?'. THIS BOOK IS FOR YOU,
MAY IT GIVE YOU SOME WELL-DESERVED RELIEF.

When using kitchen appliances please always follow the manufacturer's instructions.

HQ
An imprint of HarperCollinsPublishers Ltd
1 London Bridge Street
London SE1 9GF

www.harpercollins.co.uk

HarperCollinsPublishers
1st Floor, Watermarque Building, Ringsend Road
Dublin 4, Ireland

10 9 8 7 6 5 4 3 2

First published in Great Britain by HQ
An imprint of HarperCollinsPublishers Ltd 2021

Text Copyright © Suzanne Mulholland 2021

Suzanne Mulholland asserts the moral right to be
identified as the author of this work. A catalogue
record for this book is available from the British
Library.

ISBN 978-0-00-837324-5

Our policy is to use papers that are natural, renewable
and recyclable products and made from wood grown
in sustainable forests. The logging and manufacturing
processes conform to the legal environmental
regulations of the country of origin.

For more information visit:
www.harpercollins.co.uk/green

Photography: Haraala Hamilton
Food styling: Sam Dixon, Rosie French
  & Rosie Ramsden
Prop styling: Sarah Birks
Design & Art Direction: Georgina Hewitt
Editor: Nira Begum
Editorial Director: Kate Fox
Project Editor: Daniel Hurst

Printed and bound in Italy by Rotolito S.p.A

Suzanne Mulholland

The
BATCH
LADY

HEALTHY FAMILY
FAVOURITES

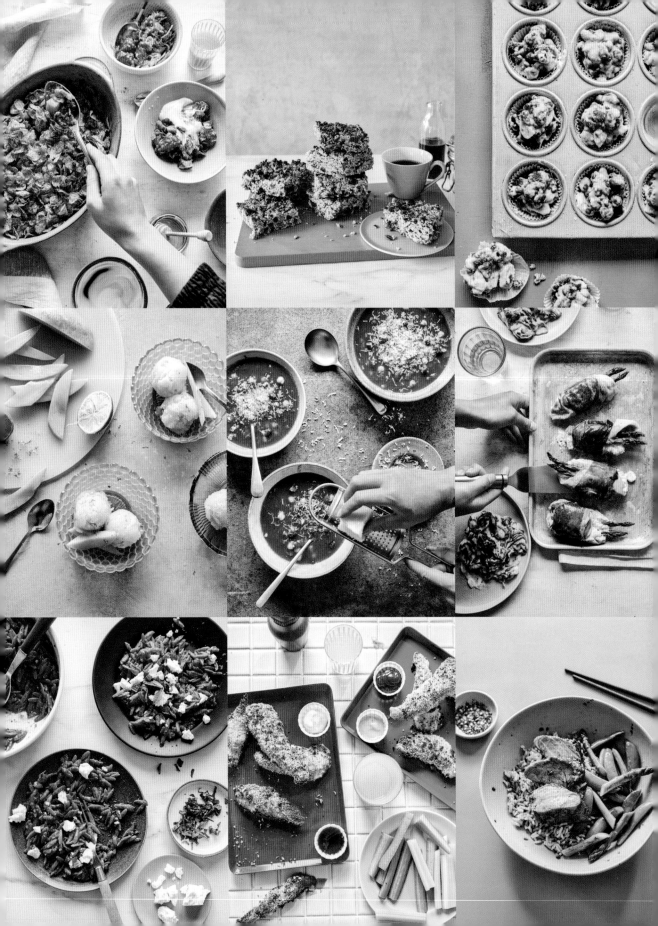

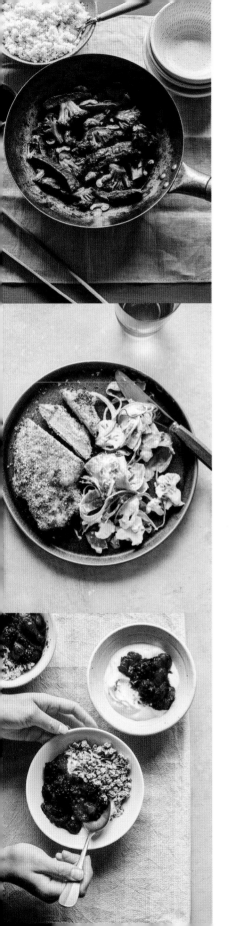

CONTENTS

WELCOME!

Or, for those who know me from my first cookbook, *The Batch Lady*, 'Welcome Back!'. Either way, whether you're a seasoned batcher who is familiar with my method or someone just dipping their toe into the world of batching for the first time, I'm thrilled to have you! And, for those new batchers, 'Hello and welcome to the world of batching – I promise it's going to revolutionise your time spent in the kitchen!'

So, a second cookbook! Who knew? I loved writing *The Batch Lady*, although as it was my first book, I was very nervous to see if people understood the concept and enjoyed the recipes. The good news is that I shouldn't have been worried and it's been amazing to see all the photos, messages and emails being sent in by everyone who has been 'getting their batch on' and telling me how much more time they have to do the things they love now that they're not shackled to the kitchen night after night.

My first book was packed full of hearty recipes that were sure to be hits with the whole family. The focus was on filling your freezer (and your belly!) with tasty food that could be on the table with as little fuss as possible. So, what's different this time round? I've kept the focus on family cooking at the heart of this book and, as before, each meal serves 4–6 and can be scaled up or down to suit the size of your household. (Plus, if you do end up with extra, that's just another meal that can be on standby in the freezer to save you cooking on another night!)

The one key difference is that these recipes have more of a focus on health. When putting food on the table for my kids, making sure that I am providing a balanced plate of food is always at the front of my mind, but as a mother and wife who's responsible for getting a family meal on the table, I am often pulled between trying to feed everyone in the house the same thing and trying to eat healthily. My children, who seem to grow taller by the day, need a nutritionally dense diet containing a good range of healthy fats. My husband and I, both in our mid 40s, can't match their metabolisms, so need to keep more of an eye on what we eat. With that in mind, the recipes in this book offer the same comforting family favourites, but with twists and tricks to make them just that little bit healthier.

Each recipe contains both 'family' and 'lighter' serving suggestions, so you can easily cater for everyone sitting around the table. While the kids might opt for rice and naan bread with their curry, the adults might prefer cauliflower rice and a dollop of yoghurt instead. Elsewhere, I've made simple substitutions to ingredients and methods of cooking that won't impact on taste or nutritional value, but are kinder on calories; for example, baking instead of frying or using turkey mince instead of beef.

If you are watching your calories, I have included a breakdown of the calorie and carbohydrate content of each meal at the top of page, so that you can easily factor those in when planning your meals. In this way, I hope that you can cater for your entire family and rest assured that, as well as being tasty, everyone is getting a well-balanced plate of food that ticks all the boxes for their individual nutritional needs.

Over the last year, I have tested these recipes night after night and have truly loved the headspace and freedom of knowing that I can eat a healthy, calorie-controlled diet, while also feeding the whole family a meal that gives them everything they want and need. I no longer have to worry about cooking two separate meals, and with the power of batching, I can have it all ready-made in advance of the week ahead to free-up my precious evenings to do the stuff I really enjoy.

As life gets ever busier, it can be hard to find time for the things that really count. As many of us deal with busy schedules, mounting work stress or feel the pull of the purse strings, planning our weekly meals can feel like an impossible task. My hope is that this book will take all that stress away with meals that are economical, waste-free, healthy, can be made ahead and, most importantly, taste great.

Believe in the batch!

Suzanne

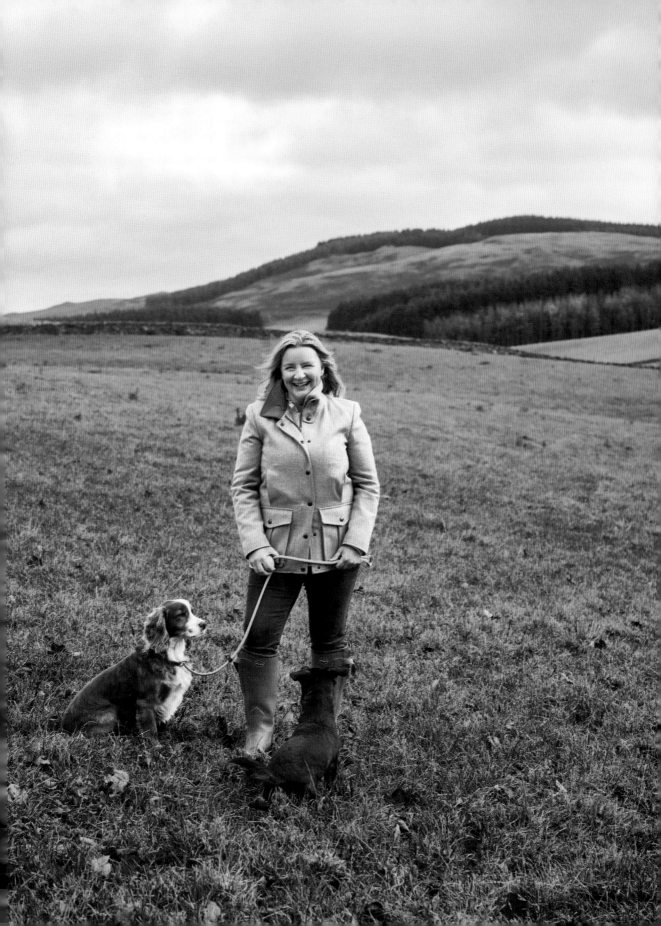

BATCH YOURSELF HEALTHY

To people who have never batch-cooked before, planning your meals ahead and cooking in large quantities can seem like a lot of work, but the truth is that cooking in this way is a massive time-saver. With this book, you have the added benefit of knowing that the food you are preparing is also healthy, balanced and ticking all of the nutritional boxes for you and your family, which will give you back both time and headspace to spend on the things you love.

THE BENEFITS OF BATCHING

Batching is, quite simply, the act of making more than one meal at a time. It's a great way of saving time and money and you don't need to have any specialist equipment, or even a large freezer. My first book, *The Batch Lady*, focussed on batch cooking family favourites, and this book follows many of the same principles, however, this time I have kept health at the front of my mind when planning the recipes.

For many of us, life is a juggling act, and planning what we are going to cook in the evening is just one of many balls that we are trying to keep in the air at any one time. As a parent, with multiple diaries to keep track of, just knowing who is going to be sat around the dinner table from day to day can seem an impossible task. And catering for different appetites and dietary requirements on top of that can quickly push you to

overload. The good news is that following my method and batch cooking your meals will free up your mental load and mean that you always have a freezer full of delicious and nutritious home-cooked meals ready to access whenever you need them.

I like to sit down at the beginning of the week and plan my meals, regardless of whether they're being made from fresh, using up what I already have ready to go in the freezer or even when I'm giving myself a night off and ordering a pizza or a curry. Once I have my plan, I can do all my shopping and spend an hour or two doing the bulk of my prep and cooking for the week. Once that's done, mealtimes are a doddle and I don't have to spend any more of my precious time worrying about what I am going to cook when. Sounds good? Let's get started.

THE RECIPES

As with all my recipes, those in this book are simple and easy to follow. They are split into chapters on Breakfasts, Light Meals, Fakeaways, Weeknights, Weekend Feasts, Sides & Sauces, and Desserts.

Where my recipes differ slightly to those in a 'traditional' recipe book is that each recipe contains different instructions depending on if you want to cook the recipe to serve now, prepare it for the freezer to eat on another day or are reheating it from frozen. This

might sound complicated, but it couldn't be simpler. Simply follow the numbered method as far as you can and then jump to whichever of the three columns at the bottom of the page matches what you want to do. If you are cooking it to serve, just follow the 'To Cook' instructions, if freezing, jump to 'To Freeze', and so on.

These are designed to be family meals serving 4–6 people, and I have always kept the whole family in mind when writing the recipes. Where dishes contain spice, I have always kept it on the milder end of the spectrum, so as not to blow any tiny tastebuds! If you're a family of spice lovers, simply adjust the seasoning to suit your tastes.

Because this a book of family cooking, another factor that I always have tried to consider is cost. You'll notice, for example, that I use a lot of turkey mince in these recipes, as opposed to beef or lamb. Turkey is a brilliant sub to make because it is both cheaper, leaner and lower in fat than other types of mince. Plus, once it's cooked into a tasty chilli or Bolognese, no one will notice the difference.

VEGETARIAN RECIPES

One of the things I get asked for a lot by followers on my social media channels is more vegetarian recipes. Many people have also said that they struggle with feeding the vegetarians in their house because their family is made up of a mix of vegetarians and omnivores. Making two meals to cater for different diets is a huge amount of extra work, so I have tried to include veggie meals that even the most determined carnivores would be happy to eat. All of the vegetarian recipes in this book are marked with a green 'V' symbol in the top corner, so are easy to identify.

The other thing to note is that many of these recipes can easily be adapted to suit a vegetarian diet by subbing in, for example, a plant-based mince instead of meat or using veggie stock instead of chicken. Even if you and your family aren't vegetarian, do give some of the veggie recipes a try as they are some of my favourite in the book.

WORKING IN PAIRS

Just like my first book, all of the recipes in this book have been put into pairs. These are dishes that lend themselves to being cooked at the same time, as they have similar ingredients or methods. In many of the recipes you will see a coloured bar running through the method. These bars give instructions on how to jump between the two recipes if you are making them both together. If, for example, a sauce on one recipe needs to bubble away for 10 minutes, that might be the perfect time to hop over to the second recipe and get it started. This is a great time-saving way of making two meals at once, and often means that you can make two meals in the time it would otherwise take you to make just one. If you want to make the meals in isolation, then that's totally fine, too – just skip past the instructions in the coloured bars when working through the recipe.

NO-COOK MEALS

Do you ever rush into the supermarket looking for a fast-fix dinner and pick up one of those little foil trays with, say, two stuffed raw chicken breasts wrapped in bacon? While these can be a tasty and quick solution to an empty fridge, they are often expensive, especially if you are feeding more than two people. The 'no-cook' recipes in this book are my version of these, but they are far cheaper to make than to buy!

The benefit of these recipes, especially if making them to store in the freezer, is that all you need to do is put all of the uncooked ingredients together in a freezer bag, then freeze and you have a ready-assembled meal prepared for another day.

These recipes are easy to spot as there is often no numbered method in the recipe itself, just the 'To Cook, To Freeze, To Cook from Frozen' instructions at the bottom of the page. This isn't a mistake – it's just because the dish is so simple to prepare that you don't need to do any actual cooking before it goes in the freezer! I often pair a 'no-cook' meal with a more complicated recipe, so you can quickly assemble one while the other is bubbling away. These are also the perfect place to start for anyone with mobility issues or who is heavily pregnant, as they can be made sitting at the kitchen table.

DOUBLE BUBBLE!

If you are going to make one, then you may as well make two! Once you've got the hang of using my method to make two meals at one time, the next step is to double the volume of the recipes you are making, so that at the end of your cooking time you will have four family meals ready for the fridge or freezer. Doing this generally only adds 5 minutes extra time to your cook, so is a great way of maximising your time and filling your freezer in the process! Equally, if you're not cooking for a family, you can easily halve the recipes in the book and put one portion in the freezer for another day.

LIGHTER SERVE VS FAMILY SERVE

In order to make it as simple as possible to feed the whole family the same meal, I have kept each main recipe relatively light and given two options for sides. This means that if you're trying to count the calories but want to give the kids something more substantial, you can easily make one main meal and switch up the side dishes so that your plate of food is just a little bit lighter.

As an example, the Low-Fat Chicken Goujons (p.126) gives the following options:

Lighter Serve: Green leafy salad and Low-Fat Caesar Dressing (p.211)

Family Serve: Piri-Piri Sweet Potato Chips (p.205) and peas

HOW LOW CAN YOU GO?

When deciding on the definition of 'healthy' for this book, I had to weigh up who was going to be sat around the dinner table eating these meals. This is family cooking, so it was important to me that it didn't read like a diet book. Rather than focussing on just calories or fat content, I have tried to design the meals so that they are nutritionally balanced and provide everything a growing child needs and satisfies their appetite. That said, I was also aware that some people cooking from this book will be watching their weight, which is why I made the decision to include the amount of calories and sugar at the top of each recipe. These figures are per portion and include the main meal, but not any side dishes. I have also made some changes to the types of ingredients used in the recipes. These are small changes that will never be noticed in the final dish, but that make a big difference in terms of lightening the nutritional load for each recipe. For example, swapping out oil for low-calorie cooking spray or low-fat margarine for butter, and using low-fat cheese and yoghurt, and low-sodium stock throughout. These are easy changes to swap back, so just do what feels right for you and your family. Your meal, your choice.

THREE WAYS WITH...

Just like my last book, within the chapters you will find features titled 'Three Ways With...' This is where I show you how to take one basic recipe and serve it three different ways. There are some recipes that lend themselves really well to being adapted in this way, for example the Sweetcorn Fritters on page 63. These can be enjoyed with eggs and bacon for breakfast or dressed up with avocado, crème fraîche and sriracha sauce and served for lunch. In this way, one basic recipe becomes three different meals, all of which feel fresh and different. This is a great way of making a big batch of one type of food and keeping the whole family interested every time you serve it!

MY BATCH COMMANDMENTS

When planning your food for the week, follow these rules and you can't go wrong!

LIFE DOESN'T ALWAYS GO TO PLAN

Make a firm meal plan for 3–4 days of the week, then pencil in a rough outline for others. It's a good idea to leave a few nights blank for when plans change, to use up leftovers or just for those days when you fancy getting a takeaway!

THINK ABOUT MEALS IN TERMS OF TIME

And pair them up with your life plan accordingly. Busy night? Pull a fast, pre-made meal from the freezer. Lazy Sunday? Why not cook a roast?

EAT MEALS FROM YOUR FREEZER

A few nights per week so you are not always cooking from scratch.

DOUBLE UP!

Cooking double quantities often takes no extra time and gives you two full meals in the time it would take to make just one. Simply eat one on the day and store the other in the freezer.

ALLOCATE A 'FILL-YOUR-FREEZER' HOUR

Once a month when you focus on cooking meals to freeze for later. To save time, make meals that use similar ingredients. (The three for the fridge, three for the freezer sections in this book are great for this.)

GET THE FAMILY INVOLVED

Asking your family what they'd like to eat in the week ahead takes the pressure off you to come up with ideas and helps keep everyone happy!

STICK TO WHAT YOU KNOW

It's fun to try something new, but don't take on too much all at once. Add one new recipe to your repetoire each week to start branching out.

BE HONEST!

Only plan meals that you know you will make. The more 'real' you are, the better the process will work.

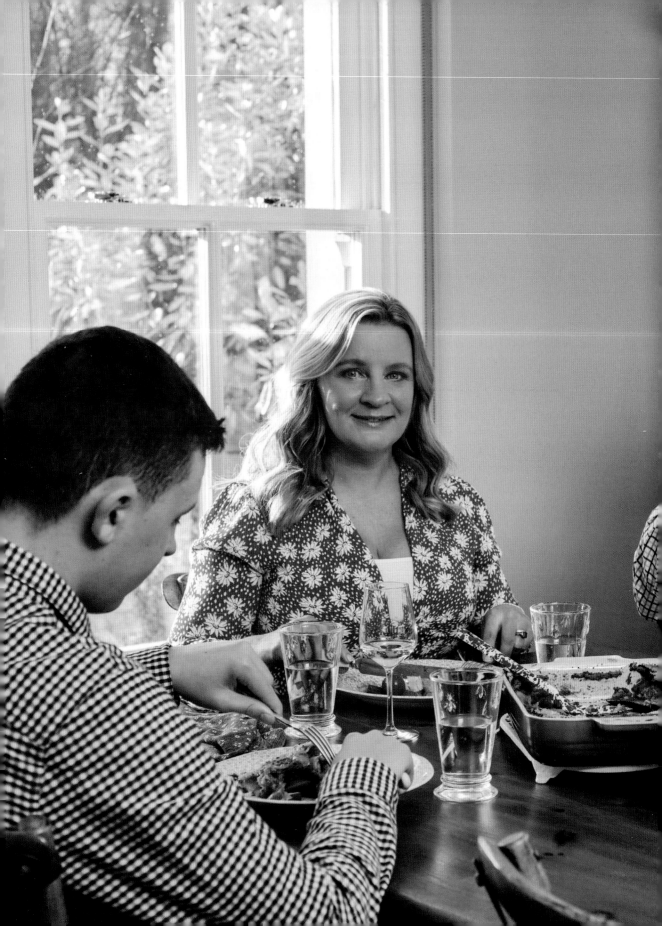

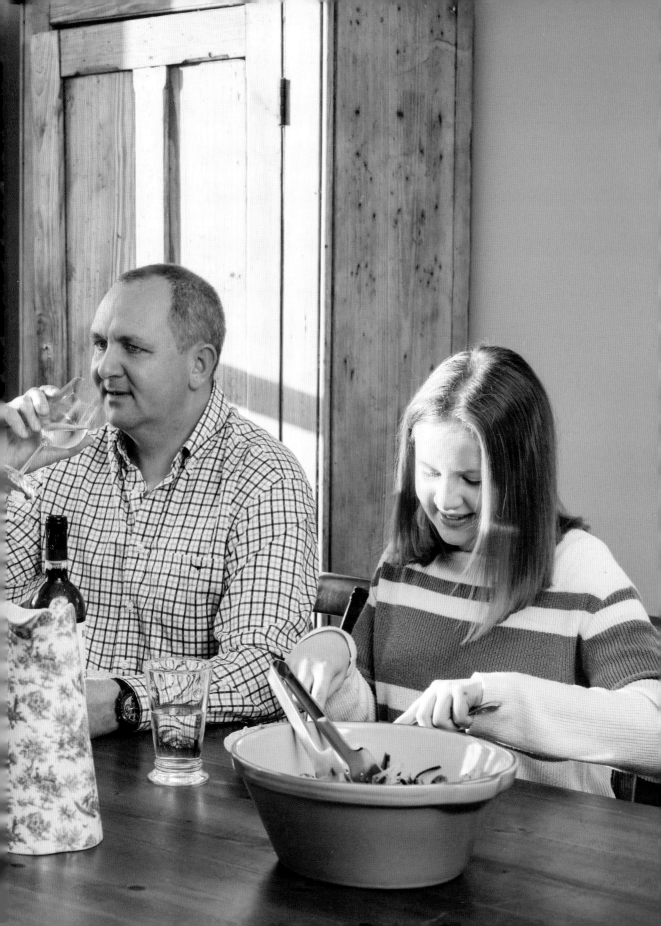

THREE FOR THE FRIDGE, THREE FOR THE FREEZER

In my previous book, I showed you how, by making meals that used similar ingredients, you could easily make 10 family meals in 1 hour. People loved this section of the book, but some of the feedback I had said that, once people had made the meals, they struggled to find the room in their freezer to fit them in. I want my books to be as accessible as possible, and not just for those with access to an enormous chest freezer, so I thought about how to adapt the method for those working a typical three-drawer freezer, and this is my solution!

Three for the fridge, three for the freezer is a way of making six family meals in 45 minutes. Three of the meals get packaged up for the freezer and the other three go into the fridge to be enjoyed in the week ahead. Each menu is made up of three different recipes, and each recipe is doubled-up to feed eight people, so simply needs to be split after cooking to make two family meals serving four people.

At the beginning of each menu you will find a shopping list that tells you exactly what you need to buy. Before going shopping, run down the list and cross out anything that you already have so that you don't end up with duplicates. It's important to note that on the shopping lists I have listed the smallest pack of each ingredient that is available to buy, not the amount actually needed in the recipe, so you may end up with a few bits leftover to make other meals.

PREPPING YOUR KITCHEN

The key to undertaking one of these mammoth cook-offs is to get really organised before you start to do any cooking. To do this, clear your kitchen counters as much as possible and give them a good clean down. You will need an area to lay out all of your ingredients as well as space to cook and portion up your meals for the fridge or freezer, so try and free-up as much space as possible.

It's also a good idea to empty your dishwasher, so you have space to deposit dirty dishes as you use them, and also empty your food-waste and general rubbish bins, so you don't find yourself having to do it when you have three meals on the go! I also like to fill my sink with hot, soapy water so that I can quickly wash any utensils that I might need to use later in the cook. Finally, make sure that you have clean tea towels, washcloths and kitchen spray to hand, so that you can wipe everything down between recipes.

Once all this done, have a read through the recipes and lay out any equipment that you'll need, so that you're not scrabbling around trying to find a saucepan or a jug at the same time as frying off your onions later. I've tried to keep the individual recipes as simple as possible, so you shouldn't need too much, but it's very useful to have everything to hand. Now the kitchen is prepared, it's time to lay out the ingredients.

SETTING OUT YOUR INGREDIENTS

On the third page of each of the three for the fridge, three for the freezer menus you will find a list of ingredients for each meal. These are ordered according to which ingredients are used first in each recipe and which recipe is prepared first across the menu. With that in mind, weigh out the ingredients for each recipe and lay them out so that the recipe you are making first is the closest to you, then the second recipe, then the third. The only exception to this is any meat or fish, which will need to stay in the fridge until you need it and any frozen ingredients that may defrost if left on the side for prolonged periods.

HOW THE RECIPES WORK

Making three different recipes at once may seem daunting, but with a little practise you'll race through the methods in no time. The recipe method for these sections contains all three dishes interwoven, so you don't have to jump between three different recipes as you cook, just follow the numbered method and you can't go wrong. As you work through, you'll see recipe headings showing you which recipe you're working on at any one time, and so you know which pile of ingredients you need to be using for that particular part of the method.

Working in this way makes the best use of your time and is the key to getting all of this done in 45 minutes. Rather than standing around and waiting for some potatoes to boil for one dish, for example, you can be getting on with the other recipes and come back to it later.

WHAT IF I WANT TO MAKE JUST ONE OF THE RECIPES?

If you want to make just one of the recipes featured in these sections, just look for the headings within the method that identify that individual recipe and ignore the rest. Do remember though that each of these recipes is doubled-up to serve 8, so you may want to halve the ingredients if you are making the dish as a single family meal.

PACKAGING UP YOUR MEALS

When prepping meals for the freezer I'm a massive fan of using reusable freezer bags (see p.23) – they prevent freezer burn, save space so that you can fit more in and simply work really well. However, when making food for the fridge, I like to use stackable plastic containers or glass dishes with lids. These pile up neatly in your fridge and you won't get any unwanted sauces dripping into your salad tray! If the dish is something that needs to go in the oven or microwave before serving, refrigerate it in a dish that can be used for that purpose, this will save on hassle and washing up later.

Whatever you put your food into, make sure to label it clearly with the name of the dish, the date it was made and, if it contains uncooked meat or fish and is going in the fridge, the use-by date of the ingredients. That way you can ensure that everything is cooked and eaten before it goes off.

When preparing food for the freezer, ensure that it is cooled to room temperature before freezing but also that it is frozen as soon as it is cool enough to do so. Food starts to deteriorate as soon as it is cooked, so the quicker it is cooled and frozen, the better.

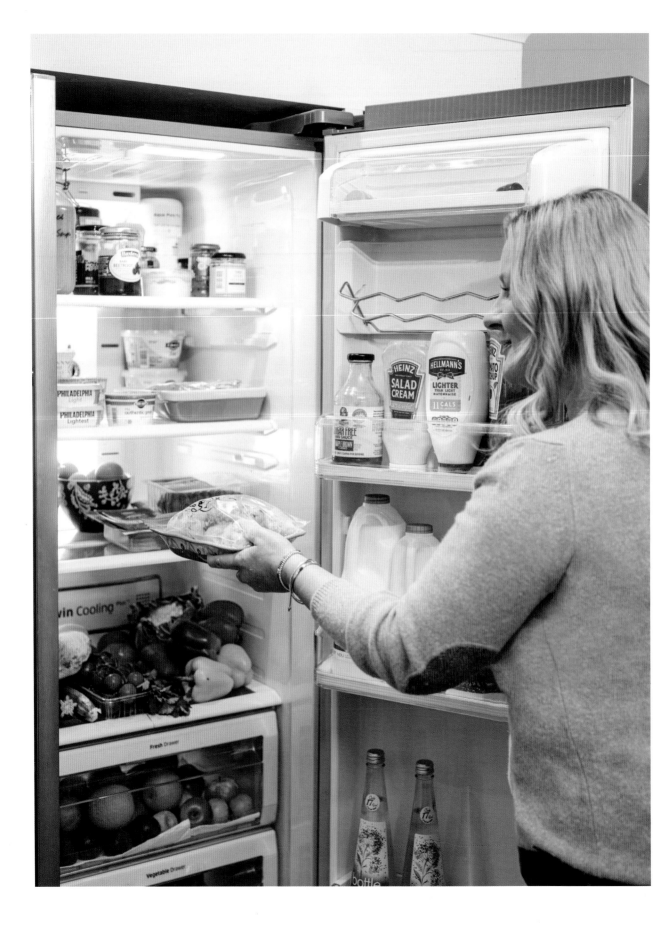

MAKING AHEAD, FREEZING & DEFROSTING

Follow the guidelines below when batching your meals for the fridge or freezer and you can't go wrong.

WHEN MAKING MEALS AHEAD FOR THE FRIDGE...

If you are making meals for the week ahead and want to store them in the fridge rather than freezing, remember that you will still have to adhere to use-by dates. If the food is cooked, it will generally keep for 2–3 days, but any 'no-cook' meals will need to be used by whatever the use-by date is on the ingredients

If you are making food at the beginning of the week to eat at the end of the week, it is best to store it in the freezer for a couple of days to ensure optimum freshness, then simply defrost in the fridge overnight the evening before you want to serve the meal.

WHEN PREPARING FOOD FOR THE FREEZER...

When you are preparing meals to be frozen and used later, ensure that all of the ingredients that you use are both fresh and in-date. Meals that have been pre-cooked need to be left to cool down to room temperature before freezing, but frozen as soon as they are cool enough to do so.

If you are making multiple recipes at once, remember to wash your hands regularly when moving from one recipe to the next to avoid any cross-contamination. Also, wash down the kitchen surfaces and clean any chopping boards and utensils before using them to make another dish. This is not only more hygienic but also saves on washing up at the end of your batching session.

When putting multiple bags of food in the freezer, try and spread them out rather than placing them all together. If you freeze a large pile of bags together at the same time, the centre bags in the stack will take far longer to freeze and the food will start to deteriorate, so it is best to spread them throughout your freezer.

WHEN DEFROSTING FOOD...

Remembering to defrost your food the day before you want to serve it can be tricky, so make it easy by setting a reminder on your phone each night at 6pm and you will always be organised. For recipes that need to be defrosted before cooking this can be done in numerous ways.

IN THE FRIDGE

Current guidelines recommend defrosting food in the fridge overnight. It is best to put defrosting food in a dish to catch any water run-off. Defrosting in your fridge can take a long time, especially if you have frozen something in a large container. With this in mind, I like to combine this method with the water method, on the following page.

IN COLD WATER

Make sure that the container or bag your frozen food is stored in is watertight, then place it in a basin of cold water (never use hot!). Doing this speeds up the defrosting process rapidly and is great for those nights that you've forgotten to take anything out of the freezer.

IN THE MICROWAVE

Most microwaves have specific defrosting programmes, so simply follow the manufacturer's guidelines for your specific model, remembering to stir your food from time to time as it defrosts.

COOKING STRAIGHT FROM THE FREEZER

For those days when you're home from work and don't have the time or energy to cook something from scratch, below is a list of recipes from this book that can be cooked directly from frozen. All reheated meals should reach a temperature of 74°C/165°F and be piping hot before serving.

DISHES THAT CAN BE COOKED FROM FROZEN

Banana Pancakes (p.34)

Beetroot & Feta Orzotto (p.182)

Bombay Potatoes (p.196)

Cauliflower Rice (p.203)

Courgette Fritters (p.62)

Chipotle Turkey Meatballs (p.147)

Creamy Tomato & Red Pepper Soup (p.54)

Creamy Salmon & Pea Parcels (p.168)

Fajita-Spiced Chicken Schnitzel (p.127)

Harissa Cauliflower Traybake (p.137)

Kedgeree (p.72)

Lamb Koftas (p.90)

Light-And-Easy Naan Breads (p.208)

Light-And-Easy Paprika Flatbreads (p.209)

Low-Fat Chicken Goujons (p.126)

Moroccan Vegetable & Chorizo Soup (p.69)

Mushroom Stroganoff (p.164)

Paprika Hasselback Potatoes (p.197)

Piri-Piri Sweet Potato Chips (p.205)

Pork Schnitzel (p.123)

Rhubarb & Strawberry Compote (p.46)

Salmon, Pea & Leek Frittata (p.73)

Skin-On Chips (p.204)

Spiced Cauliflower Steaks (p.136)

Spicy Turkey Burgers (p.141)

Stewed Apple & Blackberry Compote (p.47)

Sweetcorn Fritters (p.63)

Turkey & Orzo Soup (p.58)

Turkey Keema Matar (p.101)

Turkey 'Shepherd's' Pie (p.40)

Turkey Tagine (p.178)

Turkey Taco Boats (p.59)

White Turkey Chilli (p.146)

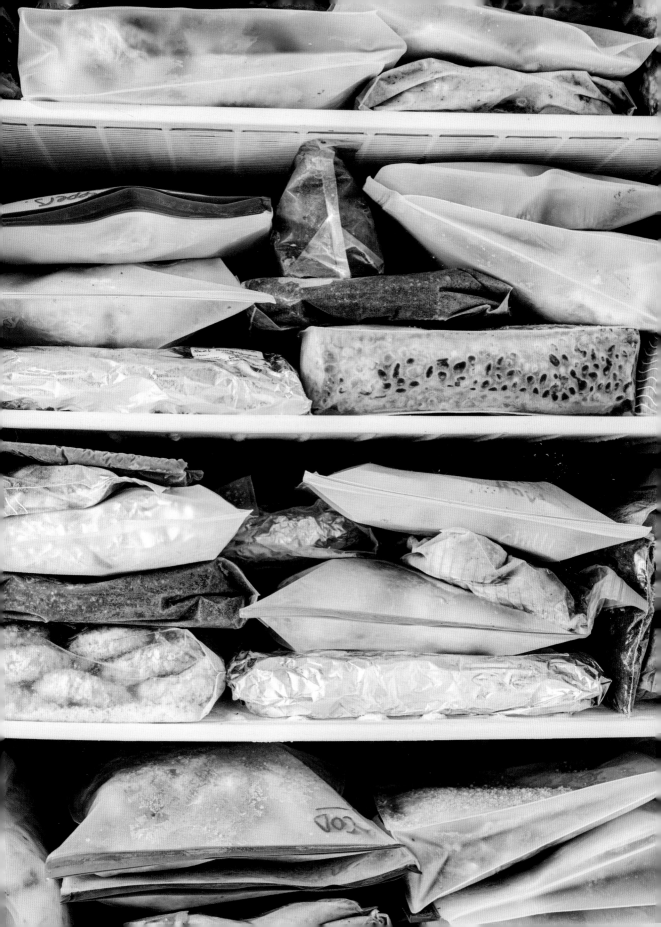

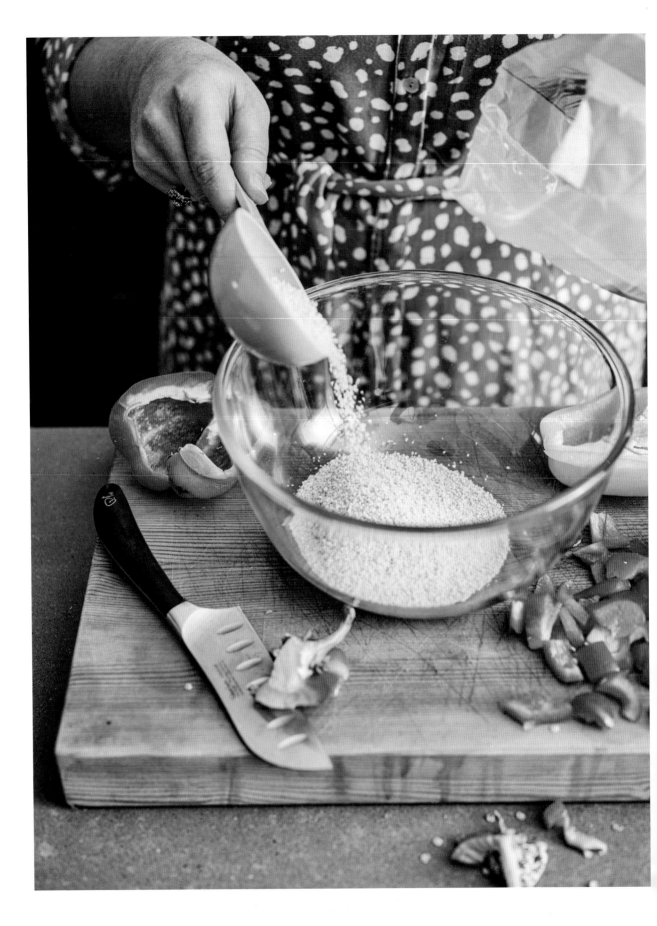

BATCHING EQUIPMENT

Batch cooking is all about making meals in the shortest amount of time, and there are a few tools that can help maximise your time and get your food packaged and in the freezer quickly. The good news is that most of them are cheap, easy to come by and you may have them in your kitchen already. If you struggle to find anything listed, do check out the shop on my website, where I sell many of these items.

MEASURING CUPS

Using cups is the quickest way of measuring ingredients, and when it comes to batching, speed is key! You'll see that I list cup measurements first in all of my recipes, although there are also gram measurements for those who prefer it. When using cups the most important thing to know is that you can't just grab any mug from your cupboard. A 'cup' is a standard measure (see the table below), so it's worth investing in a set if you're planning on batching regularly. These look like a large set of measuring spoons and generally come in full cups, ½ cups, ⅓ cups and ¼ cups. Once you have your set, simply scoop up your ingredients and level off the top – much easier than weighing everything out on a set of scales!

CUP MEASUREMENTS

1 cup	240ml	16 tablespoons	½ cup	120ml	8 tablespoons
¾ cup	180ml	12 tablespoons	⅓ cup	80ml	5½tablespoons
⅔ cup	160ml	11 tablespoons	¼ cup	60ml	4 tablespoons

PORTIONING WITH CUPS

If you have decided to double-up on a recipe, it can be difficult to visualise just how much food you've made and how many people it will serve. Cups can help with this, as you can divide the food between several freezer bags equally (depending on how many times you have scaled the base recipe up). As a general rule, one cup of 'scoopable' food (such as a curry or a stew) will feed one person. For children who are under 10, use ½ a cup per child.

LARGE, NON-STICK COOKING POTS

If you're going to be doubling-up your recipes then you will need large pots to cook them in. I recommend getting at least two, so you can have more than one meal on the go at once. When looking to invest in pots, choose non-stick versions that are oven-safe – that way you can transfer your meals from the stove to the oven without having to spend time decanting them into another dish first. Also, if you are watching your calorie intake, using a non-stick pan cuts down on the amount of oil you need to use at the beginning of a recipe. A good-quality pot should last for 10–15 years, so is a long-term investment.

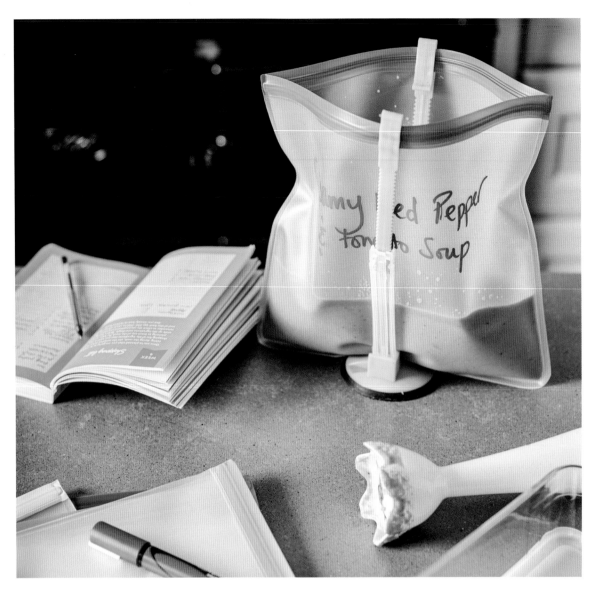

LARGE MICROWAVEABLE GLASS BOWLS

These handy bowls can be used for mixing and combining ingredients, but are also good for defrosting food in the microwave or placing over a pan of hot water, if needed.

FREEZER BAGS

Freezer bags are brilliant for saving space in your deep-freeze and for preventing freezer burn. They also allow you to freeze your food flat, so you can stack them side-by-side in the freezer and make the most of the space available. In this way you will end up with a library of meals, much like a stack of books all neatly arranged in your freezer (see p.19). When deciding on which bags to use, there are three types to choose from.

SEALABLE PLASTIC FREEZER BAGS

These are the most common variety and can easily be found in supermarkets and corner shops. They come in a variety of sizes and, crucially for the environment, it is becoming more common for them to be able to be washed and reused several times before throwing away. They are flexible and transparent, so are easy to use. However, they generally only last for a handful of uses before they need to be replaced.

PEVA BAGS

This is a new type of freezer bag that is a more easily reusable alternative to traditional plastic freezer bags. They are made of food-grade PEVA (polyethylene vinyl acetate), which means they can be used to store food in the freezer or in the fridge. They are generally very flexible and offer the same benefits of plastic food bags, but have the added bonus that they can be washed out and reused up to 350 times. The downside to them is that they are made of a non-chlorinated vinyl that cannot be heated, put in the dishwasher or microwave. This also mean that hot food should be left to cool before adding to the bags.

SILICONE BAGS

Silicone food bags are the most expensive option, but they are high quality, are the best for the environment and the safest to use. You can heat them up, add them to your dishwasher or even cook in them. They are often less flexible than other types of freezer bag and are opaque rather than fully see-through. If you are going to be batching regularly, these are a good investment for both you and the environment.

FREEZER-TO-OVEN BAKING DISHES

These brilliant ovenproof glass dishes come with plastic lids for when you store food in the fridge or freezer. The best thing about them is that they can go straight from the freezer to the oven, which makes them perfect for dishes such as a shepherd's pie or lasagne, that you may want to cook directly from frozen.

MARKERS AND CHALK PENS

It's always a good idea to label everything that goes into your fridge or freezer. If you've made up 'no-cook' meals (see p.9) for the fridge, then you want to make sure that you label with the use-by date of any ingredients, and when putting meals in the freezer, labelling avoids finding that you have a UFO (unidentified frozen object) when it comes to cooking it later. Marker pens are fine, but can be difficult to remove from reusable tubs and bags. Chalk pens make a great alternative as they can easily be washed off with soap and water, freeing you up to use a freezer bag or Tupperware container time and again.

FREESTANDING OR HANDHELD BLENDER

Some of the recipes in this book call for a freestanding or handheld stick blender. These are great for making things like smoothies, soups and sauces. They are relatively cheap, great time-savers and yield brilliant results, so are a worthwhile investment.

THE HEALTHY LARDER

A well-stocked larder or storecupboard is the backbone of successful batching and, once you've been doing this for a while, you'll find that you have many of the ingredients for my recipes to hand and just need to top-up on the fresh dairy, meat and veg rather than doing a full shop. With all of my recipes I try and use ingredients that are easy to get hold of and won't break the bank, so you may well have a lot of this stuff in your cupboards already, especially if you cook from my previous book. One difference in this book is that I have subbed in some lower-calorie, lower-fat alternatives to keep the recipes as lean as possible. Again, these are easy to get hold of and won't break the bank.

PASTA, RICE & PULSES

couscous
dried pasta (orzo, macaroni, wholewheat lasagne sheets and wholewheat spaghetti)
noodles
oats
panko breadcrumbs
quinoa
red lentils
rice (basmati, brown basmati and risotto)

CANS, JARS & BOTTLES

chickpeas
chopped tomatoes
cornflour
Dijon mustard
hoisin sauce
jarred capers
low-sodium soy sauce
olive oil
passata
red kidney beans
red wine vinegar
reduced-fat coconut milk
sesame oil
sundried tomatoes
sweet chilli sauce
sweetcorn
tikka masala spice paste
white wine vinegar
wholegrain mustard
Worcestershire sauce

HERBS & SPICES

Cajun spice
chilli flakes
chilli powder
Chinese 5 spice
curry powder
dried dill
dried oregano
dried rosemary
dried thyme
fajita spice mix
garlic granules
ground cinnamon
ground coriander
ground cumin
paprika (smoked and unsmoked)
piri-piri seasoning
sesame seeds
tagine spice mix

SAUCES, STOCKS & PASTES

chipotle paste
harissa paste
lemongrass paste
low-sodium stock cubes (beef, chicken and vegetable)
reduced-salt-and-sugar tomato ketchup
tomato purée

SWEET BITS & BAKING

agave nectar
baking powder
cashew nuts
cornflakes
dried apricots
flour (plain, self-raising and wholemeal)
light evaporated milk
low-fat granola
maple syrup
pumpkin seeds
raisins
reduced-fat digestive biscuits
runny honey
shop-bought meringue nests
sugar (caster and icing)
vanilla extract

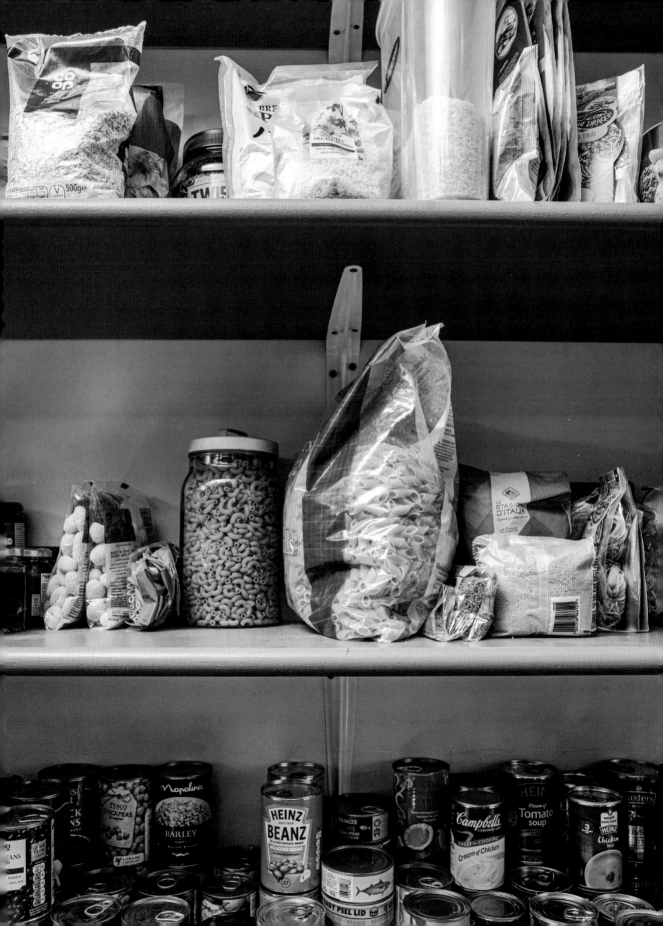

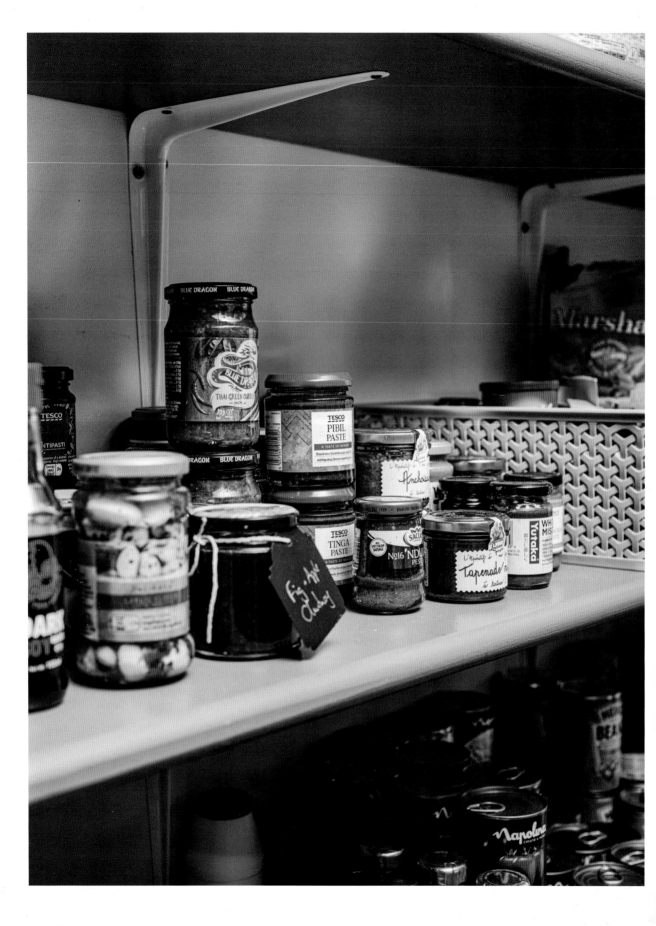

SKINNY SUBSTITUTIONS

The recipes in this book are generally made using traditional, rather than specific low-calorie or 'diet', ingredients. However, if you do want to reduce the calories of any of the meals further you could substitute ingredients with the lighter alternatives in the table below.

INGREDIENT	LOWER CALORIE ALTERNATIVE
sugar	light agave nectar, stevia, light maple syrup, honey, sugar free syrup
butter	low-fat margarine or spread
cheese	low-fat cheese
oil	low-calorie cooking spray
chorizo	turkey bacon
mayonnaise	0% fat yoghurt, extra-light mayonnaise
milk	skimmed milk, soy milk, almond milk, oat milk
bread/tortilla wraps	low-fat wraps
ketchup	reduced-salt-and-sugar tomato ketchup, tomato purée
rice	Cauliflower Rice (p.203)
pasta	spiralised courgette
ice cream	frozen yoghurt

FROZEN, CHOPPED VEGETABLES

Frozen vegetables are picked at their best, then washed, peeled, chopped and flash-frozen to retain all their nutrients. What's not to love?! Still not convinced? Here are some other benefits if using pre-prepared, frozen veg.

All of the work is done for you! Using frozen veg is perfect for batch cooking as you don't have to peel or chop vegetables, which is a massive time-saver.

There's no waste. We've all been guilty of finding soggy, past-their-best veg languishing at the bottom of the veg drawer in the fridge. Frozen veg avoids this unnecessary waste. Simply use what you need and put the rest back in the freezer for another day.

The one down-side of frozen veg is the plastic packaging that it comes in, but as we become more switched on to the environmental impact of the food that we buy, the good news is that this is changing. The frozen-food industry has pledged to go plastic-free and is looking into ways to change the packaging it uses. One change that we can already see is the zip-lock bag that some freezer veg comes in. Don't throw these away, as they can be reused once you've used up all the veg.

WANT TO USE FRESH INSTEAD OF FROZEN?

If you prefer to use fresh fruit and vegetables instead of frozen for the recipes in this book, then you can. Use the table below to work out how much of a fresh ingredient you will need to substitute for its frozen counterpart. Do bear in mind that the cooking times for fresh will be different and adjust them accordingly.

INGREDIENT	FROZEN	FRESH
chopped onions	1 cup	1 onion, finely chopped
chopped red onions	1 cup	1 red onion, finely chopped
mixed sliced peppers	1 cup	1 pepper, deseeded and sliced
chopped spinach	2 cubes	½ bag fresh spinach, chopped
sliced carrots	1 cup	2 carrots, peeled and sliced
sweet potato chunks	1 cup	1 medium sweet potato, chopped
sliced leeks	1 cup	1 small leek, sliced
raspberries	1 cup	125g fresh
strawberries	1 cup	160g fresh
blueberries	1 cup	110g fresh
chopped mango	1 cup	1 mango, peeled, stoned and diced
sliced peaches	1 cup	2 peaches, peeled, stoned and sliced

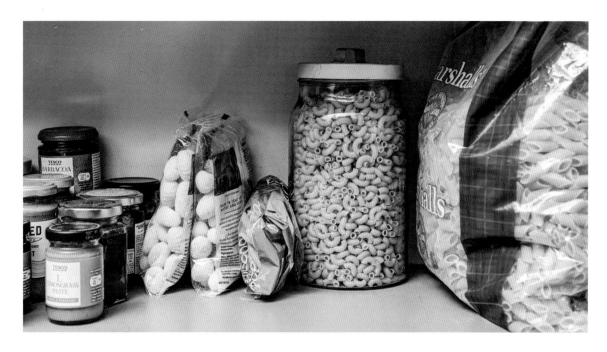

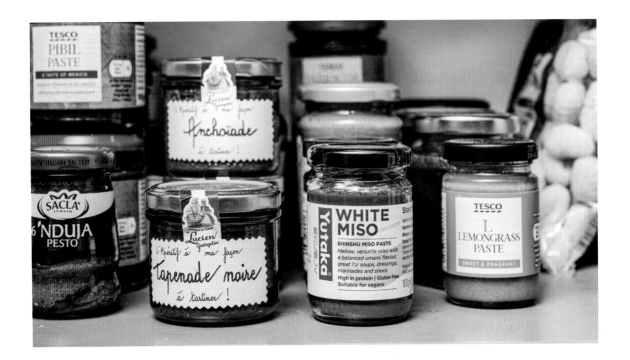

HERBS

Fresh herbs can be expensive and often don't last long. For this reason, I tend to use frozen herbs rather than fresh whenever possible. These are now readily available in most supermarkets and, much like frozen vegetables, are great for making meals fast, saving money and avoiding food waste. If you prefer to use fresh herbs, the table below gives you the difference in quantity needed between fresh, frozen, dried and puréed, so you can tailor the recipe to suit whatever you have available to you.

FROZEN HERB	FROZEN AMOUNT	FRESH EQUIVALENT	DRIED EQUIVALENT	PURÉED EQUIVALENT
frozen coriander	1 teaspoon	1 teaspoon, chopped	⅓ teaspoon	½ teaspoon
frozen parsley	1 teaspoon	1 teaspoon, chopped	⅓ teaspoon	½ teaspoon
frozen chilli	1 teaspoon	½ chilli, chopped	⅓ teaspoon	½ teaspoon
frozen basil	1 teaspoon	1 teaspoon, chopped	⅓ teaspoon	½ teaspoon
frozen rosemary	1 teaspoon	1 teaspoon, chopped	⅓ teaspoon	½ teaspoon
frozen chopped ginger	1 teaspoon	2.5cm (1in) piece, peeled and grated	⅓ teaspoon	½ teaspoon
frozen thyme	1 teaspoon	1 teaspoon, chopped	⅓ teaspoon	½ teaspoon
frozen chopped garlic	1 teaspoon	1 clove, crushed	½ teaspoon	½ teaspoon

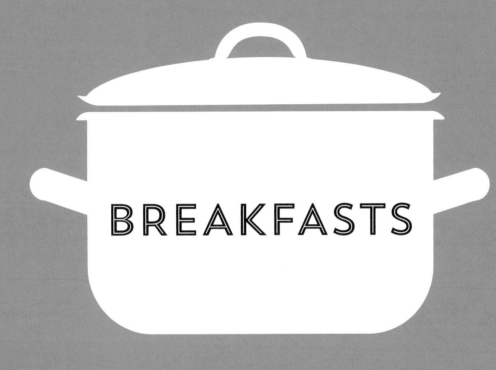

BREAKFASTS

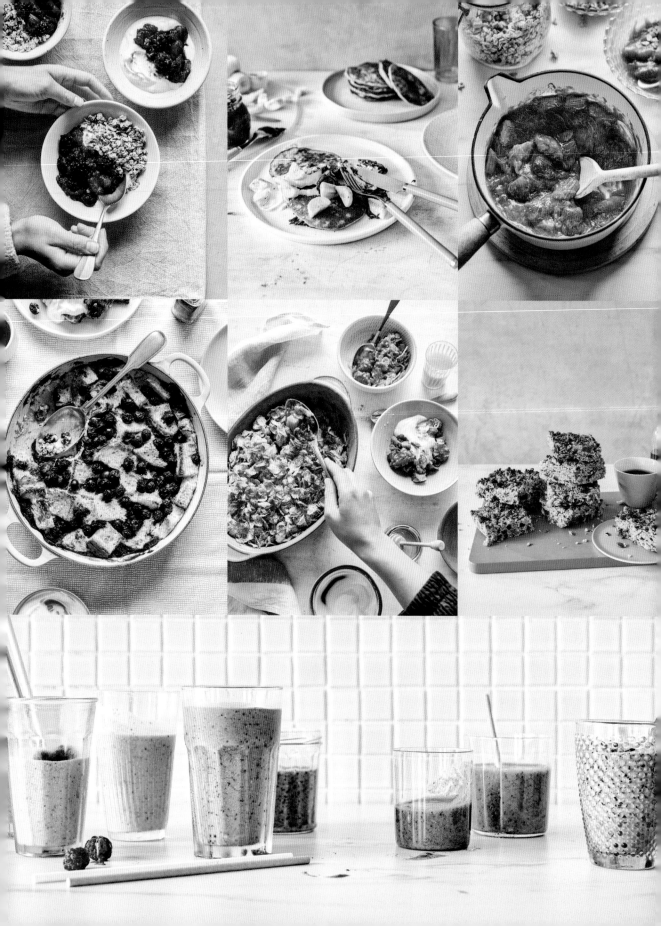

BREAKFASTS

A healthy breakfast will set you up for the day and keep you and your family satisfied and focussed all the way to lunchtime, but busy mornings can often mean that there isn't time for anything more than a quick bowl of cereal as you race through the kitchen on the way out the door. The good news is that with a few of the recipes from this chapter stored away in the freezer, even mid-week breakfasts can be a bit more special.

Healthy grab-and-go smoothie bags or Banana Pancakes that can be popped into the toaster straight from frozen (p.34) mean that breakfast in a hurry needn't be boring and, for lazy weekend breakfasts, indulgent-but-light treats, such as my Blueberry French Toast Bake (p.35) or Apple & Plum Cornflake Bake (p.43) feel really celebratory without being heavy. If you're looking for more weekend brunch dishes, there are also recipes elsewhere in this book that can be dressed up with eggs or yoghurt for a weekend-worthy treat; try the Shakshuka (p.55), Courgette Fritters (p.62), Sweetcorn Fritters (p.63) or Kedgeree (p.72).

BANANA PANCAKES

PREP: 5 MINS **COOK:** 5-10 MINS **SERVES:** 4 **SUGAR:** 14G **KCAL:** 160

These delicious pancakes can be frozen and then quickly reheated in the toaster, making them a great healthy option for busy school mornings. I like to make a big batch of these, so why not double the recipe and fill the freezer?

3 bananas
2 eggs, beaten
½ cup (60g) wholemeal plain flour
½ tsp ground cinnamon
1 tsp baking powder
splash of milk (optional)
low-calorie cooking spray

To serve

Lighter Serve: Low-fat natural yoghurt and sliced banana
Family Serve: Yoghurt, hazelnut and chocolate spread and sliced banana

1 Peel the bananas and add to a large bowl, mashing against the side with a fork until smooth. Add the eggs, flour, cinnamon and baking powder and whisk to a smooth batter. If the mixture is too thick, add a splash of milk to loosen slightly. Set aside for 10 minutes to rest.

> If you are also making the Blueberry French Toast Bake, assemble this now while the batter is resting.

2 Spray a non-stick frying pan with low-calorie cooking spray and place over a medium heat. Once the pan is hot, add a ladleful of batter to the pan and cook for 2–3 minutes, until golden underneath, then flip and cook the other side. Remove from the pan and set aside on a rack to cool while you make the rest of the pancakes in the same way.

TO SERVE

The pancakes are now ready to serve with your choice of toppings.

TO FREEZE

Leave the pancakes on the rack to cool to room temperature, then transfer to a large, labelled freezer bag and freeze flat for up to 3 months.

TO REHEAT FROM FROZEN

These can be defrosted and reheated quickly in the pan, or cooked from frozen by putting them in the toaster until fully defrosted and piping hot all of the way through.

BLUEBERRY FRENCH TOAST BAKE

PREP: 10 MINS **COOK:** 30–40 MINS **SERVES:** 4 **SUGAR:** 16G **KCAL:** 467

This breakfast feels really celebratory and weekend worth and is sure to be a hit with adults and children alike, but is actually low in both sugar and fat. Any leftover blueberries can be frozen and used when serving the Banana Pancakes (opposite), or just enjoyed with a bowl of low-fat yoghurt and a handful of a granola for another delicious, easy-win breakfast.

8 slices bread (approx. 420g), cut into 2.5cm (1in) squares
1½ cups (195g) frozen or fresh blueberries
5 eggs
2½ cups (600ml) semi-skimmed milk
1 tsp vanilla extract
1 tsp ground cinnamon
2 tbsp maple syrup

To serve
Lighter Serve: Low-fat natural yoghurt and blueberries spooned over
Family Serve: Yoghurt, maple syrup and extra blueberries spooned over

1 Scatter the squares of bread over the base of a large baking dish and spoon the blueberries over the top.
2 Crack the eggs into a large bowl and beat together with the milk, vanilla extract, cinnamon and maple syrup.

TO COOK

Scatter the squares of bread over the base of large baking dish and spoon the blueberries over the top. Pour over the egg and milk mixture and set aside to soak for 30 minutes. Once soaked, transfer the dish to an oven preheated to 180°C/350°F/gas mark 4 for 30–40 minutes, until golden and well risen.

TO FREEZE

Layer the bread and blueberries in a large, labelled freezer bag and pour over the egg and milk mixture. Carefully seal the bag, expelling any excess air and freeze flat for up to 3 months.

TO COOK FROM FROZEN

Remove from the freezer and defrost in the fridge, ideally overnight. Pour the mixture into a large baking dish and cook as described left, until golden and well risen.

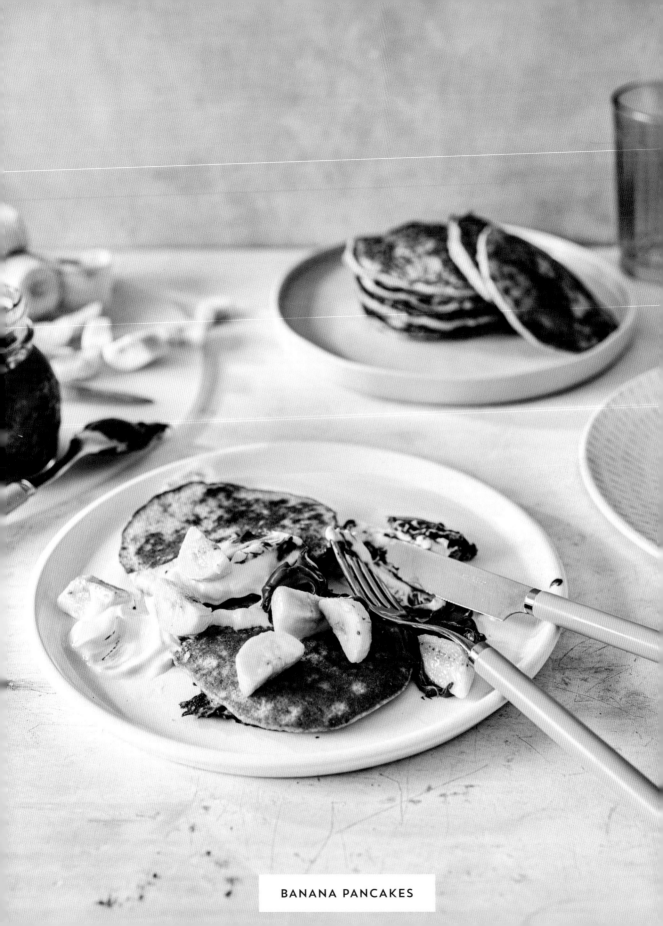

BANANA PANCAKES

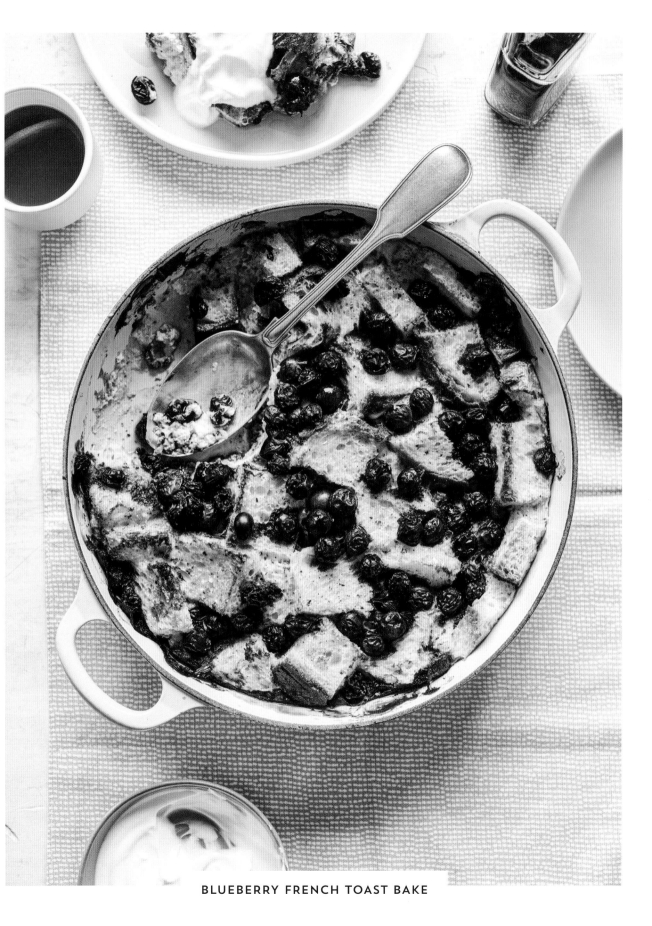

BLUEBERRY FRENCH TOAST BAKE

BANANA & STRAWBERRY SMOOTHIES

PREP: 5 MINS **MAKES:** 4 **SUGAR:** 29G **KCAL:** 240

These wonderfully healthy smoothie bags are a great way to start the day. Simply grab the bag out of the freezer, add some milk and blitz for a quick and nutritious brekkie! I have offered four different variations here, so why not fill your freezer so that you can have something that feels fresh and different every day?

2 cups (300g) frozen strawberries
2 large bananas, sliced
½ cup (110g) low-fat Greek
 yoghurt
½ cup (50g) porridge oats

To serve
1 tbsp honey
2½ cups (600ml) water or milk

TO FREEZE

You can freeze this in 1 large batch making 4 smoothies, or split the mixture into 4 separate freezer bags for individual portions before freezing. Either way, put the frozen strawberries, sliced bananas, yoghurt and porridge oats in a labelled freezer bag (or bags) and freeze flat for up to 3 months.

TO SERVE FROM FROZEN

Remove the bag from the freezer and transfer the contents to a freestanding blender. Add the honey and water or milk to the blender (reducing the amounts to scant ⅔ cup (150ml) of milk and ¾ teaspoon of honey if you are making an individual portion) and blend until smooth. If the smoothie is too thick, add a little more water or milk and blend again. Pour into glasses and serve.

SUPERFOOD SMOOTHIES

PREP: 2 MINS **MAKES:** 4 **SUGAR:** 23G **KCAL:** 219

2 cups (260g) frozen blueberries
2 large bananas, sliced
2 handfuls fresh spinach
½ cup (110g) low-fat Greek
 yoghurt
½ cup (50g) porridge oats

To serve
1 tbsp honey
2½ cups (600ml) water or milk

TO FREEZE

You can freeze this in 1 large batch making 4 smoothies, or split the mixture into 4 separate freezer bags for individual portions before freezing. Either way, put the frozen blueberries, sliced bananas, spinach, yoghurt and porridge oats in a labelled freezer bag (or bags) and freeze flat for up to 3 months.

TO SERVE FROM FROZEN

Remove the bag from the freezer and transfer the contents to a freestanding blender. Add the honey and water or milk to the blender (reducing the amounts to scant ⅔ cup (150ml) of milk and ¾ teaspoon of honey if you are making an individual portion) and blend until smooth. If it is too thick, add a little more water or milk. Serve.

BERRY BLAST SMOOTHIES

PREP: 2 MINS **MAKES:** 4 **SUGAR:** 16G **KCAL:** 179

1 cup (150g) frozen strawberries
1 cup (130g) frozen blueberries
1 cup (115g) frozen raspberries
½ cup (110g) low-fat Greek
  yoghurt
½ cup (50g) porridge oats

To serve
1 tbsp honey
2½ cups (600ml) water or milk

TO FREEZE

You can freeze this in 1 large batch making 4 smoothies, or split the mixture into 4 separate freezer bags for individual portions before freezing. Either way, put the frozen fruit, yoghurt and porridge oats in a labelled freezer bag (or bags) and freeze flat for up to 3 months.

TO SERVE FROM FROZEN

Remove the bag from the freezer and transfer the contents to a freestanding blender. Add the honey and water or milk to the blender (reducing the amounts to scant ⅔ cup (150ml) of milk and ¾ teaspoon of honey if you are making an individual portion) and blend until smooth. If the smoothie is too thick, add a little more water or milk and blend again. Pour into glasses and serve.

SUPER GREENS SMOOTHIES

PREP: 2 MINS **MAKES:** 4 **SUGAR:** 18G **KCAL:** 93

3 kiwis, peeled and roughly
  chopped
1 cup (100g) grapes
2 handfuls fresh spinach
2 bananas, sliced

To serve
2½ cups (600ml) water

TO FREEZE

You can freeze this in 1 large batch making 4 smoothies, or split the mixture into 4 separate freezer bags for individual portions before freezing. Either way, put the chopped kiwis, grapes, spinach and sliced bananas in a labelled freezer bag (or bags) and freeze flat for up to 3 months.

TO SERVE FROM FROZEN

Remove the bag from the freezer and transfer the contents to a freestanding blender. Add the water to the blender (reducing the amount to scant ⅔ cup (150ml) if you are making an individual portion) and blend until smooth. If the smoothie is too thick, add a little more water and blend again. Pour into glasses and serve.

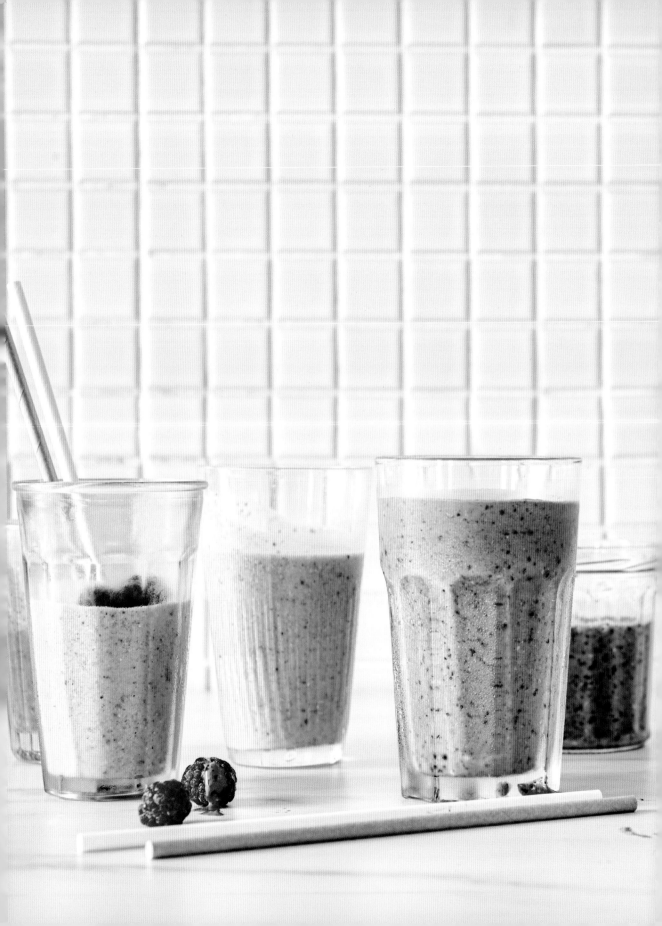

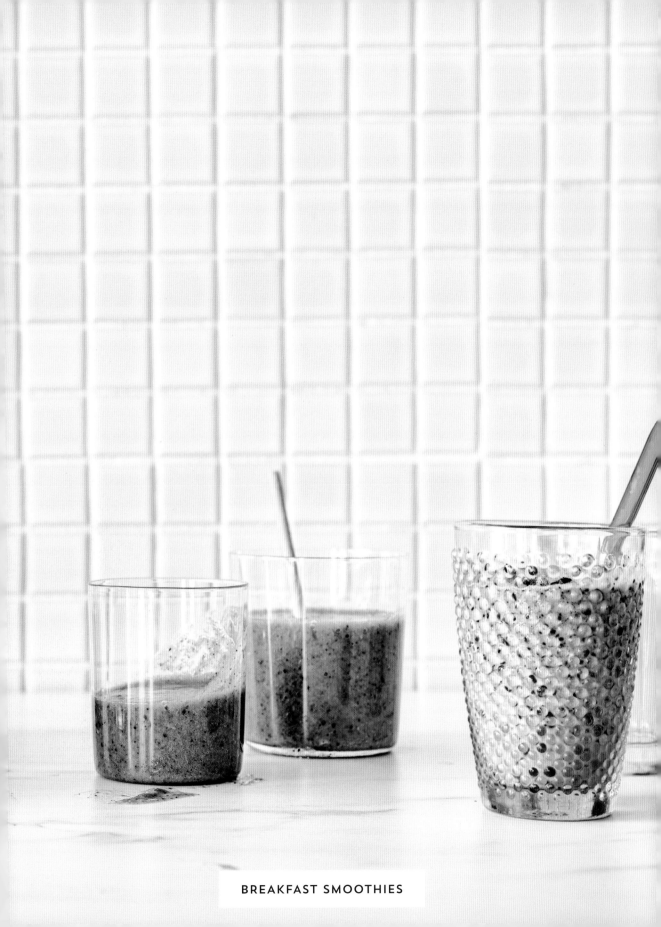

BREAKFAST SMOOTHIES

HEALTHY FLAPJACK

PREP: 10 MINS **COOK:** 15-18 MINS **MAKES:** 12 FLAPJACKS **SUGAR:** 14G **KCAL:** 215

Packed full of good stuff, these make a brilliant grab-and-go breakfast for those days when even cereal is too much of a stretch! They defrost at room temperature in about an hour, so are great additions to the kids' lunchboxes and, if added straight from the freezer, will keep everything else nice and chilled, too.

low-calorie cooking spray
⅔ cup (100g) golden syrup
100g low-fat margarine
1 heaped tbsp smooth peanut
  butter
2½ cups (250g) rolled oats
½ cup (65g) pumpkin seeds
½ cup (70g) raisins or sultanas
12 dried apricots, finely chopped
1 large banana, mashed with a fork
1 egg, beaten

1 Preheat the oven to 180°C/350°F/gas mark 4. Spray a 30 x 20cm (12 x 8in) baking tin with low-calorie cooking spray and line with baking parchment.
2 Put the golden syrup, margarine and peanut butter in a large pan over a low heat and cook, stirring, until melted. Remove from the heat.
3 Add the oats, pumpkin seeds, raisins or sultanas, dried apricots, mashed banana and the beaten egg to the pan and stir until everything is well combined.
4 Tip the mixture into the prepared baking tin and press down firmly into an even layer. Transfer to the oven and cook for 15–18 minutes, until firm and golden. Set aside to cool to room temperature.

> If you are also making the Apple & Plum Cornflake Bake, cook the fruit for that now while the flapjack is in the oven.

5 Set aside to cool to room temperature, then carefully remove from the tin and slice into 12 equal-sized pieces.

TO SERVE

The flapjacks are now ready to slice and serve.

TO FREEZE

Slice the flapjacks, then transfer them to a large, labelled freezer bag or airtight container and freeze flat for up to 3 months.

TO SERVE FROM FROZEN

Simply remove as many flapjacks as you need from the freezer and set aside to defrost at room temperature. This will take around 1 hour.

APPLE & PLUM CORNFLAKE BAKE

PREP: 10 MINS **COOK:** 20–30 MINS **SERVES:** 4 **SUGAR:** 33G **KCAL:** 301

This is a wonderful, warming breakfast for chilly autumn and winter days when a bowl of cereal simply isn't going to cut it. It might seem like an elaborate dish to serve on a busy morning, but if you make the fruit mixture and keep it in the freezer, you can simply defrost it overnight and have this on the table in the same time that it would take you to rustle up a bowl of porridge.

8 plums, pitted and roughly
  chopped
2 medium cooking apples, cored,
  peeled and roughly chopped
2 tbsp runny honey
1 tsp ground cinnamon
1 tsp vanilla extract
For the topping:
¼ cup (50g) low-fat margarine
2½ cups (110g) cornflakes
1 tbsp runny honey

To serve
Lighter Serve: Low-fat natural
yoghurt
Family Serve: Yoghurt and honey

1 Put the plums, apples, honey, cinnamon, vanilla extract and
   2 tablespoons of boiling water in saucepan over a medium heat
   and cook, stirring occasionally, for 10–12 minutes, until the fruit
   has softened and started to break down.

TO COOK

Transfer the fruit mixture to a large baking dish and set aside. Put the low-fat spread in a small bowl and microwave in 10-second bursts, until melted. Put the cornflakes and honey in a large bowl, pour over the melted spread and stir to combine. Spoon the cornflake mixture over the top of the fruit in an even layer, then transfer the dish to an oven preheated to 180°C/350°F/gas mark 4 for 10 minutes, until the topping is just starting to turn a deep golden colour. Spoon into bowls and serve hot.

TO FREEZE

Set the fruit mixture aside to cool to room temperature, then spoon into a large, labelled freezer bag and freeze flat for up to 3 months.

TO COOK FROM FROZEN

Remove the bag containing the fruit mixture from the freezer and leave to defrost, ideally in the fridge overnight. Once defrosted, transfer the mixture to a large baking dish and make the topping mixture as described in the *To Cook* section, left. Spoon the cornflake mixture over the top of the fruit in an even layer, then transfer the dish to an oven preheated to 180°C/350°F/gas mark 4 for 15–18 minutes, until the fruit is piping hot and the topping is a deep golden colour. Spoon into bowls and serve.

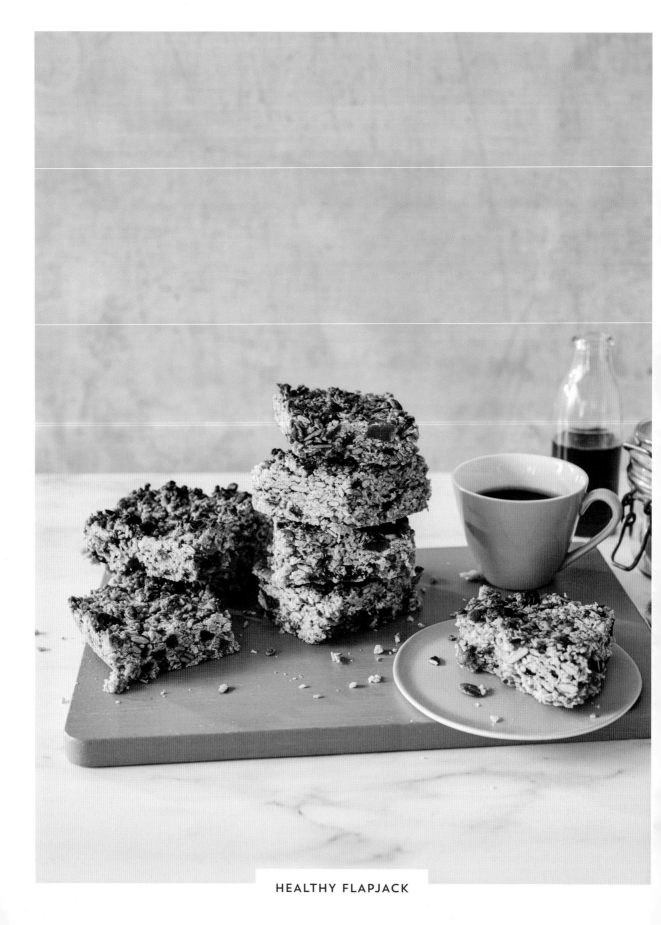

HEALTHY FLAPJACK

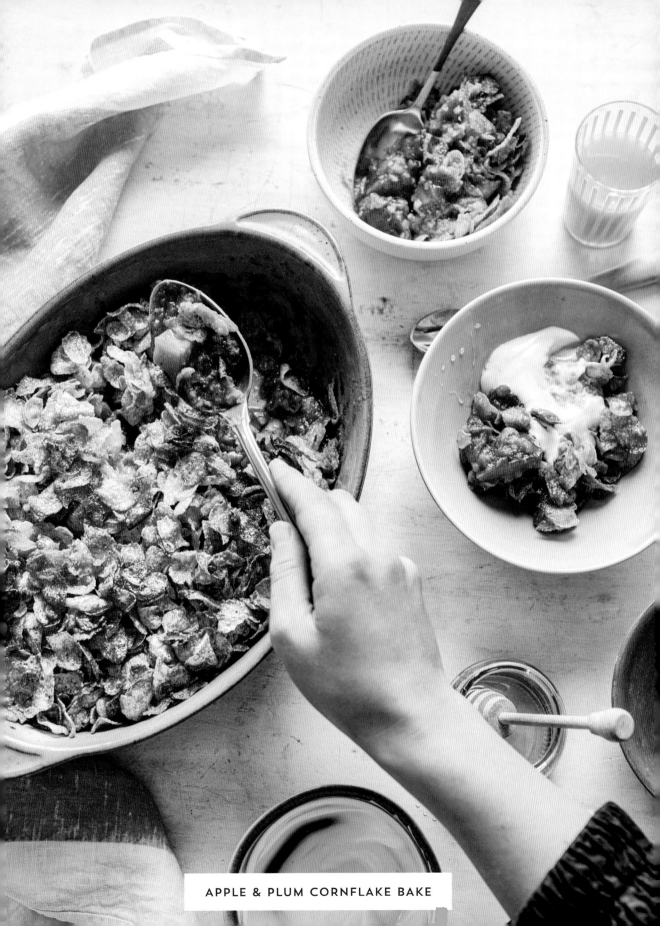

APPLE & PLUM CORNFLAKE BAKE

RHUBARB & STRAWBERRY COMPOTE

PREP: 5 MINS **COOK:** 10 MINS **SERVES:** 4 **SUGAR:** 13G **KCAL:** 77

These two compote recipes are packed with fruity flavour and provide a wonderful way to dress up a mundane breakfast and make it feel fresh and vibrant. The natural sweetness of the fruit means that these are equally at home on the dessert table as at breakfast and a bowl of compote and low-fat yoghurt is a great, guilt-free way to curb those late-night sugar cravings.

3 stalks fresh rhubarb (approx. 280g), chopped into 2cm (¾in) pieces, or same weight of frozen chunks

2 tbsp runny honey

2 cups (280g) fresh strawberries, hulled and quartered

1 tsp vanilla extract

juice of ½ lemon

To serve

Lighter Serve: Low-fat Greek yoghurt

Family Serve: Yoghurt and granola or spooned over porridge

1 Put the rhubarb and honey in a large saucepan over a medium heat with 2 tablespoons of boiling water. Bring just to the boil, then reduce the heat to a gentle simmer and leave to cook for 8 minutes, stirring occasionally, until the rhubarb has softened.

> If you are also making the Stewed Apple & Blackberry Compote, get the fruit cooking for that now.

2 Add the strawberries, vanilla extract and lemon juice to the pan, stir to combine and leave to cook for 1 minute more. Remove the pan from the heat.

TO SERVE

The compote can be served warm or cooled to room temperature. It is wonderful with yoghurt and granola or spooned into a warming bowl of porridge.

TO FREEZE

Set the pan of compote aside until cooled to room temperature, then transfer to a large, labelled freezer bag and freeze flat for up to 3 months.

TO REHEAT FROM FROZEN

The compote can be fully defrosted in the fridge or reheated from frozen. If defrosted, simply use as is or warm gently in a pan. If reheating from frozen, tip the compote into a pan with a splash of water, place over a gentle heat and warm, breaking up with a wooden spoon, until fully defrosted and piping hot all of the way through.

STEWED APPLE & BLACKBERRY COMPOTE

V

PREP: 5 MINS **COOK:** 12 MINS **SERVES:** 4 **SUGAR:** 11G **KCAL:** 63

This is a great way to dress up a bowl of yoghurt or porridge and turn a simple breakfast into something that feels special. It can be served warm or cold and, once made, will keep in a jar in the fridge for up to 5 days.

2 large cooking apples, cored, peeled and chopped
1 tbsp runny honey
1 cup (144g) fresh blackberries

To serve
Lighter Serve: Low-fat Greek yoghurt
Family Serve: Yoghurt and granola or spooned over porridge

1 Put the apples and honey in a large saucepan over a medium heat with 2 tablespoons of boiling water. Bring just to the boil, then reduce the heat to a gentle simmer and leave to cook for 8–10 minutes, stirring occasionally, until the apples have softened.
2 Add the blackberries to the pan, stir to combine and leave to cook for 2 minutes more. Remove the pan from the heat.

TO SERVE

The compote can be served warm or cooled to room temperature. It is wonderful with yoghurt and granola or spooned into a warming bowl of porridge.

TO FREEZE

Set the pan of compote aside until cooled to room temperature, then transfer to a large, labelled freezer bag and freeze flat for up to 3 months.

TO REHEAT FROM FROZEN

The compote can be fully defrosted in the fridge or reheated from frozen. If defrosted, simply use as is or warm gently in a pan. If reheating from frozen, tip the frozen compote into a pan with a splash of water, place over a gentle heat and warm, breaking up with a wooden spoon as it defrosts, until fully defrosted and piping hot all of the way through.

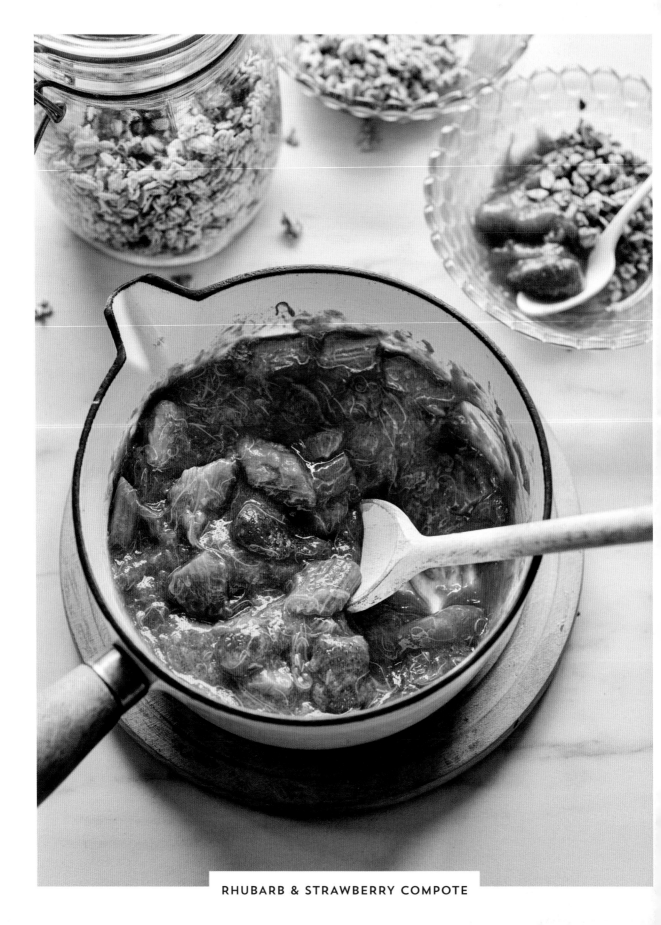

RHUBARB & STRAWBERRY COMPOTE

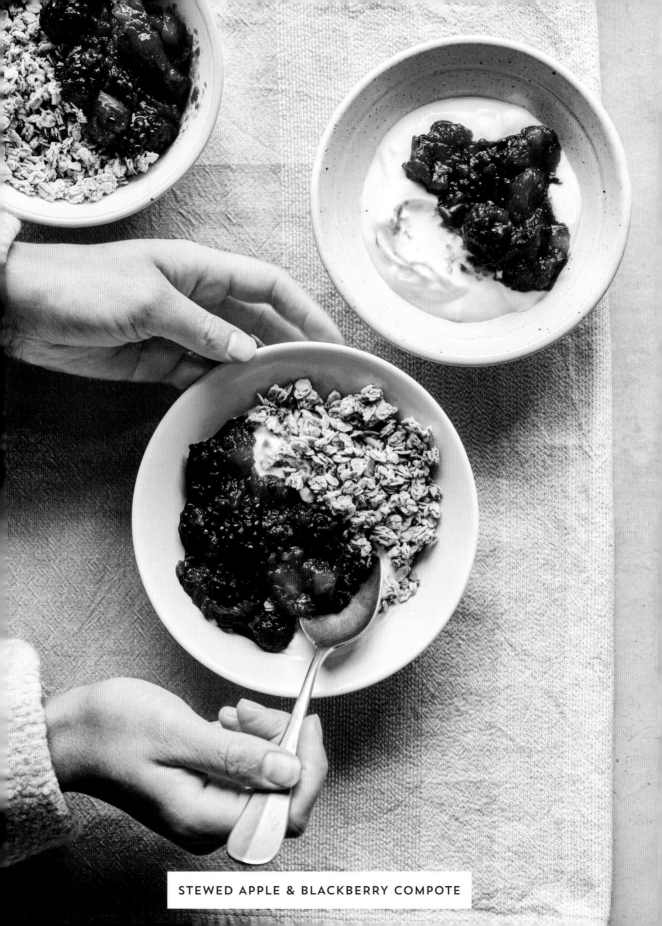

STEWED APPLE & BLACKBERRY COMPOTE

LIGHT
MEALS

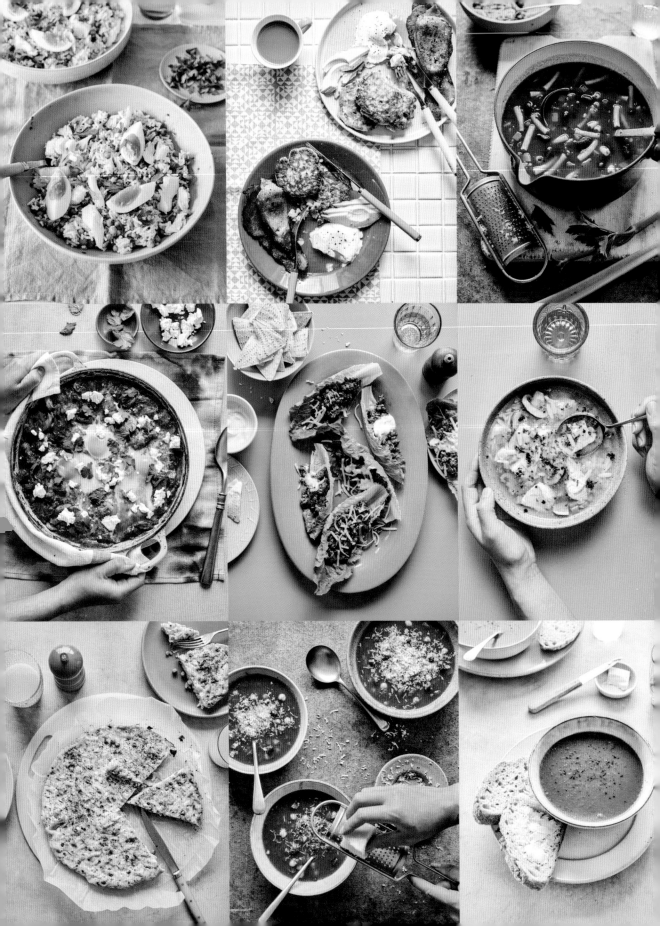

LIGHT MEALS

The recipes in this chapter make perfect lunches or are great for those days when you just want a light meal to round off the day. I'm a big fan of soups, as although light, they can also be hearty and nourishing, so you'll find a few recipes for those here, including my Turkey & Orzo Soup (p.58) and a delicately spiced Moroccan Vegetable & Chorizo Soup (p.69). My soups also have the benefit of being able to be cooked straight from frozen, so are perfect for those days when you want something tasty and homemade, but haven't made it to the shops.

Fish dishes, such as Kedgeree (p.72) and my Salmon, Pea and Leek Frittata (p.73) also feature here, as delicate fish works really well in lighter dishes and has the benefit of being wonderfully healthy. You will also find lighter takes on family classics, such as my Turkey Taco Boats (p.59), which are served in crisp lettuce cups rather than the traditional tacos.

This section also includes my first *3 for the Fridge, 3 for the Freezer* section (p.76–81), which features three flavour-packed, and all vegetarian recipes, so is a great place to start if you want to fill your fridge and freezer with some healthy and tasty options for light meals in the week ahead.

CREAMY TOMATO & RED PEPPER SOUP

PREP: 5 MINS **COOK:** 30 MINS **SERVES:** 4 **SUGAR:** 15G **KCAL:** 120

This hearty soup is easy to prepare and guaranteed to be a winner on a cold day. It can be cooked straight from the freezer, so is perfect for chilly days when you want a hug in a bowl in a hurry!

low-calorie cooking spray
1 cup (115g) frozen chopped
   onions
1 tsp frozen chopped garlic
3 red peppers, deseeded and diced
2 x 400g cans chopped tomatoes
2 cups (480ml) low-sodium
   vegetable stock
2 tbsp light cream cheese
salt and freshly ground pepper

To serve
Lighter Serve: Wholemeal pitta breads
Family Serve: Buttered sourdough bread

1 Spray a large saucepan with low-calorie cooking spray and place over a medium heat. Add the onions, garlic and peppers and cook, stirring continuously, for 2–3 minutes, until softened.
2 Add the chopped tomatoes and stock, then season to taste with salt and pepper. Bring to the boil, then reduce the heat to a gentle simmer and cook, stirring occasionally, for 25–30 minutes, until reduced and slightly thickened.

> If you are also making the Shakshuka, cook the tomato sauce for that now while the soup is cooking.

3 Once the soup has finished cooking, remove from the heat and stir through the cream cheese. Using a handheld stick blender, blend the soup until smooth, then check the seasoning.

TO SERVE

Serve the soup hot with your choice of accompaniments.

TO FREEZE

Set the soup aside to cool to room temperature, then transfer to a large, labelled freezer bag (a zip-lock bag works best for this) and freeze flat for up to 3 months.

TO REHEAT FROM FROZEN

This can be defrosted in the fridge overnight and then reheated in a pan until piping hot, or cooked from frozen. If cooking from frozen, tip the frozen soup into a large saucepan, cover with a lid and place over a low heat (you may need to break it down with a wooden spoon to get it to fit in the pan). Cook the soup, removing the lid occasionally and breaking it up with a wooden spoon as the mixture defrosts, until fully defrosted and piping hot all of the way through.

SHAKSHUKA

PREP: 10 MINS **COOK:** 25 MINS **SERVES:** 4 **SUGAR:** 17G **KCAL:** 334

This makes a wonderful lazy weekend brunch or lunch and the vibrant flavours will really set you up for the day ahead. Keep an eye on the eggs in the oven and try and remove the shakshuka just at that sweet spot when the whites are cooked but the yolks are still nice and runny. Don't worry if you do overcook them, though – the dish will still taste delicious.

1 tbsp olive oil
1 cup (115g) frozen chopped
  onions
1 tsp frozen chopped garlic
1 tsp smoked paprika
1 tsp ground cumin
2 cups (350g) frozen sliced
  peppers
2 cups (140g) white mushrooms,
  sliced
1 tbsp tomato purée
2 x 400g cans chopped tomatoes
½ tsp chilli flakes (optional)
1 tsp runny honey

To serve
4–6 eggs
100g low-fat feta cheese
small bunch fresh coriander,
  chopped

1 Add the oil to a large, stove-and-oven-safe casserole dish and place over a medium heat. Add the onions and garlic and cook, stirring continuously, for 2–3 minutes, until soft and translucent.
2 Add the smoked paprika, cumin, peppers, mushrooms, tomato purée, chopped tomatoes and chilli flakes, if using, to the pan and stir to combine. Bring to the boil, then reduce the temperature to a gentle simmer and leave to cook, stirring occasionally, for 10 minutes.

TO COOK

Remove the pan from the heat and press 4–6 dimples into the surface of the tomato mixture. Crack an egg into each dimple, then transfer the casserole dish to an oven preheated to 180°C/350°F/ gas mark 4 and cook for around 10 minutes, until the egg white is cooked through but the yolks are still runny. Crumble over the feta cheese and garnish with chopped coriander, then serve.

TO FREEZE

Remove the pan from the heat and set aside until the tomato mixture has cooled to room temperature. Transfer to a large, labelled freezer bag and freeze flat for up to 3 months.

TO COOK FROM FROZEN

Remove the tomato sauce from the freezer and leave to fully defrost in the fridge, ideally overnight. Transfer the defrosted tomato mixture to a large stove-and-oven-safe casserole dish and place over a medium heat, stirring occasionally, for around 10 minutes, until piping hot all of the way through. Continue cooking the shakshuka as per the *To Cook* instructions, left.

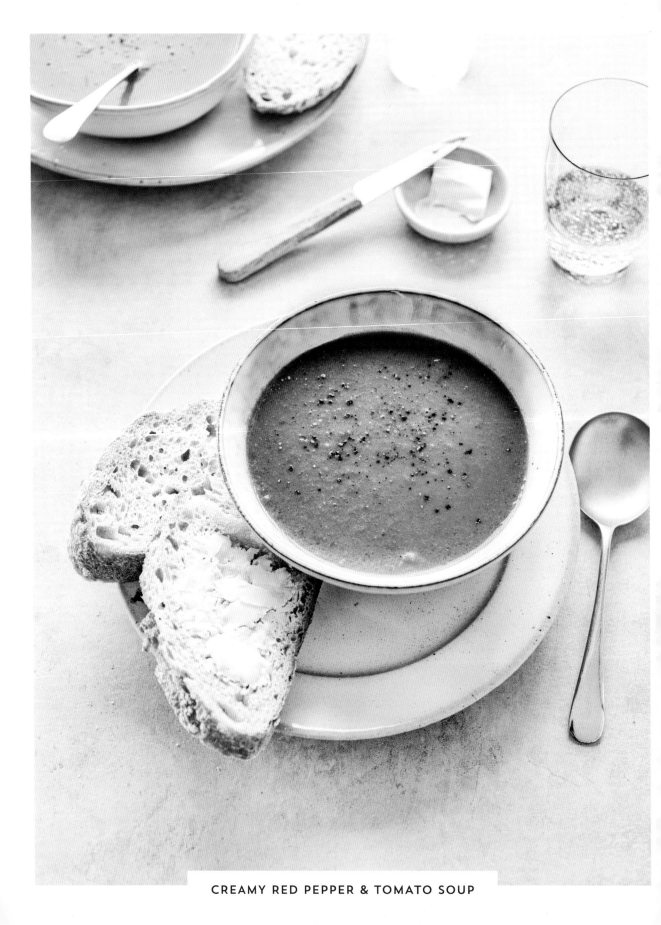

CREAMY RED PEPPER & TOMATO SOUP

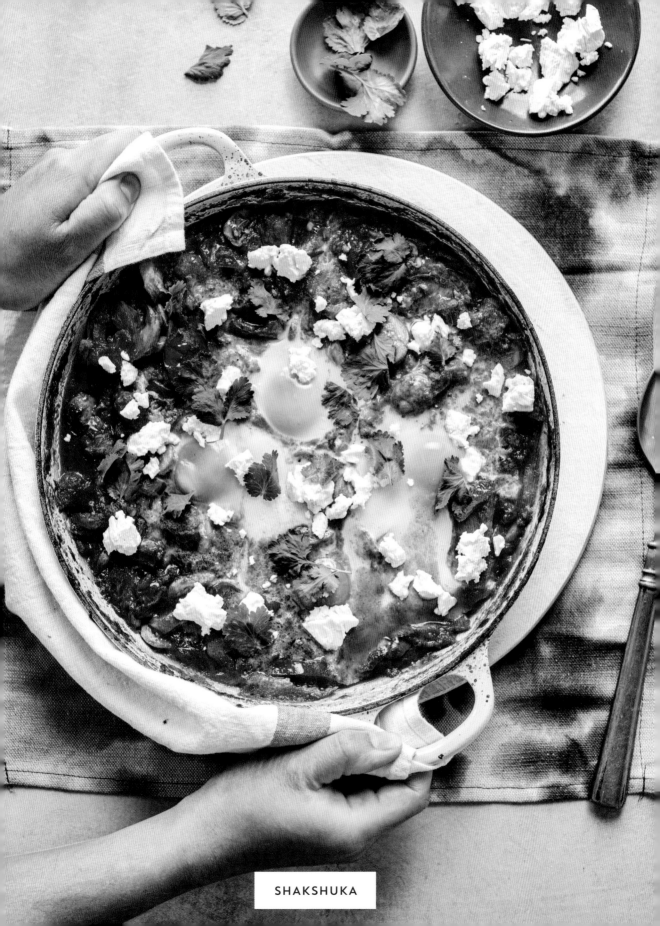

SHAKSHUKA

TURKEY & ORZO SOUP

PREP: 10 MINS **COOK:** 30 MINS **SERVES:** 4 **SUGAR:** 3.3G **KCAL:** 251

This delicious soup is perfect for a cold day when the whole family wants something hearty and warming. If you're in a rush, it can be cooked straight from the freezer, so is a great stand-by to have on hand after a chilly winter walk.

1 tbsp olive oil

3 turkey breast steaks, cut into bite-sized pieces

1 cup (115g) frozen chopped onions

1 tsp frozen chopped garlic

1 tsp frozen chopped ginger

2 sticks celery, finely chopped

1 large carrot, peeled and finely chopped

1 cup (80g) chestnut mushrooms, sliced

5 cups (1.2 litres) low-sodium chicken stock

1 bay leaf (optional)

½ cup (100g) dried orzo

1 tsp frozen chopped parsley

To serve

Lighter Serve: Wholemeal pitta breads

Family Serve: Crusty bread and butter

1 Heat the oil in a large pan over a medium heat. Once hot, add the turkey and cook, stirring, for around 5 minutes, until browned. Using a slotted spoon, transfer the turkey from the pan to a bowl and set aside, Keep the pan on the heat.

2 Add the onions, garlic, ginger, celery, carrot and mushrooms to the pan and cook, stirring, for 1 minute.

3 Add the chicken stock and bay leaf, if using, to the pan and stir to combine. Bring the mixture to the boil, then reduce the heat to a gentle simmer and leave to cook for 20 minutes to let the flavours develop.

> If you are also making the Turkey Taco Boats, start the filling mixture now while the soup is cooking.

4 After 20 minutes, add the cooked turkey back to the pan along with the orzo and parsley and stir to combine. Leave the soup to cook, stirring occasionally, for 8 minutes, until the orzo is tender. Remove the pan from the heat.

TO SERVE

The soup is now ready to be ladled into bowls and served hot with your choice of bread alongside.

TO FREEZE

Leave the soup to cool to room temperature, then ladle into a large, labelled freezer bag (a zip-lock bag works best for this) and seal, expelling any excess air as you do so. Freeze flat for up to 3 months.

TO REHEAT FROM FROZEN

This can be defrosted in the fridge overnight and then reheated in a pan until piping hot, or cooked from frozen. If cooking from frozen, tip the frozen soup into a large pan, cover with a lid and place over a low heat. Cook the soup, removing the lid occasionally and breaking it up with a wooden spoon as the mixture defrosts, until fully defrosted and piping hot all of the way through.

TURKEY TACO BOATS

PREP: 5 MINS **COOK:** 20–25 MINS **SERVES:** 4 **SUGAR:** 6.3G **KCAL:** 246

This has all of the flavour of a taco, but is served in lettuce cups for a much lighter dish. If your kids miss the crunch of the taco shells, simply crumble some tortilla chips over their portions.

low-calorie cooking spray
1 cup (115g) frozen chopped onions
2 tsp frozen chopped garlic
500g lean turkey mince
½ tsp chipotle paste
1 tsp paprika
1 tsp ground cumin
1 red pepper, deseeded and finely chopped
1 green pepper, deseeded and finely chopped
2 tbsp tomato purée
1 cup (240ml) low-sodium chicken stock
8 romaine lettuce leaves, to serve

To serve

Lighter Serve: Top with a sprinkling of low-fat, pre-grated cheese
Family Serve: Top with grated cheese, sour cream and crumbled tortilla chips

1 Spray a large, deep-sided frying pan with low-calorie cooking spray and place over a medium heat. Add the onions and garlic and cook, stirring continuously, for 2–3 minutes, until soft.
2 Add the turkey mince, breaking it up with a wooden spoon, and cook, stirring regularly, until browned.
3 Add the chipotle paste, paprika, ground cumin, chopped peppers and tomato purée and stir to combine.
4 Pour in the chicken stock and stir again. Bring the mixture to the boil, then reduce the heat to a gentle simmer and leave to cook, stirring occasionally, for 15 minutes, until the meat and peppers are tender. Remove the pan from the heat.

Make it Veggie!

For a veggie twist on this dish, swap the turkey mince with fresh or frozen plant-based mince and cook the taco filling in the same way. Plant-based mince tends to cook quicker than meat, so adjust the cooking time according to packet instructions.

TO SERVE

Divide the romaine lettuce leaves between 4 plates, then divide the turkey mixture between the leaves, using them as boats to hold the filling. Add your choice of toppings and serve.

TO FREEZE

Leave the taco filling mixture to cool to room temperature, then transfer to a large, labelled freezer bag and freeze flat for up to 3 months.

TO REHEAT FROM FROZEN

This can be defrosted in the fridge overnight and then reheated in a pan until piping hot, or cooked from frozen. If cooking from frozen, tip the frozen taco mixture into a large pan, cover with a lid and place over a low heat. Cook the mixture, breaking it up with a wooden spoon as the mixture defrosts, until it is fully defrosted and piping hot. Serve as described left.

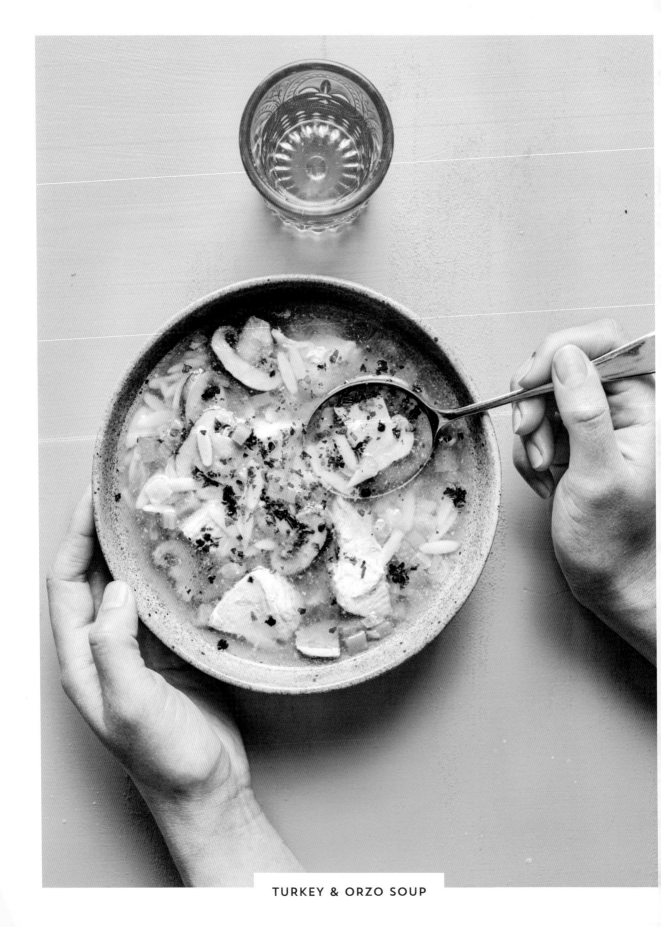

TURKEY & ORZO SOUP

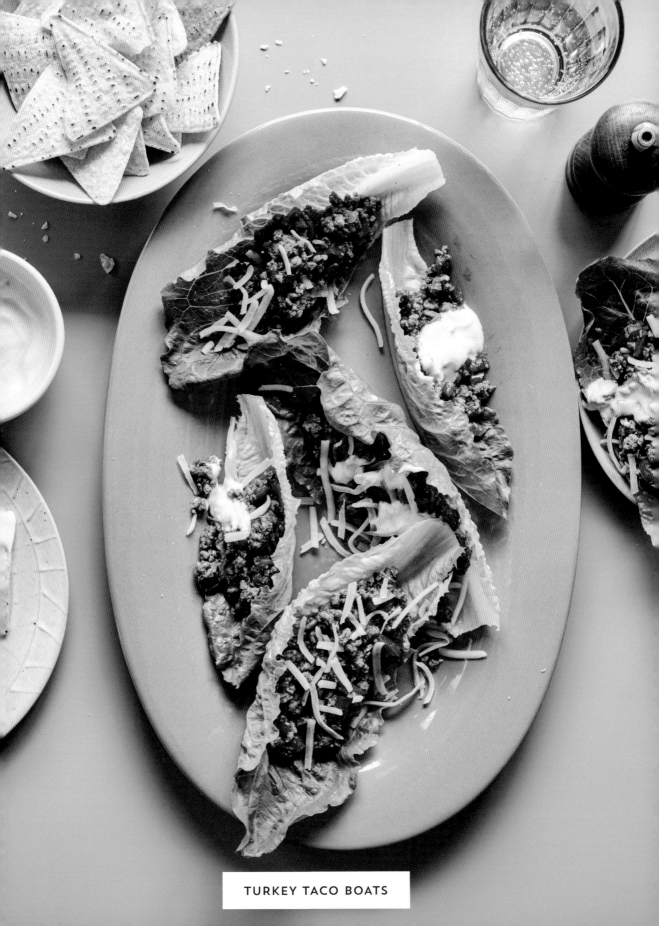

TURKEY TACO BOATS

COURGETTE FRITTERS

PREP: 8–10 MINS **COOK:** 8 MINS **SERVES:** 4 **SUGAR:** 1.9G **KCAL:** 263

These delicious fritters are perfect at any time of day and can be dressed up or down to suit. For breakfast, pair them with bacon and eggs, at lunch try them with smoked salmon and crème fraîche, or for dinner add a side of steamed kale and some Harissa Dressing (p.210). Healthy, versatile and delicious.

1 cup (110g) grated courgette
1½ cups (165g) plain flour
1 tsp baking powder
3 eggs, beaten
3 tbsp low-fat crème fraîche
5 spring onions, finely sliced
½ tsp dried mint
½ cup (120ml) milk
low-calorie cooking spray
salt and freshly ground pepper

To serve
Lighter Serve: Smoked salmon and low-fat crème fraîche
Family Serve: Crispy bacon and poached eggs

1   Lay the grated courgette on a clean tea towel, bring up the sides of the towel to enclose the courgette and squeeze and twist over the sink to remove as much liquid as possible from the courgette. This will prevent your fritters from being soggy.

2   Tip the courgette into a large mixing bowl, then add the flour, baking powder, eggs, crème fraîche, spring onions, mint, milk and a generous grinding of salt and pepper. Mix well to combine.

> If you are also making the Sweetcorn Fritters, prepare the batters for both fritters side-by-side and place two pans on the heat at the same time. That way you can cook the fritters side-by-side and minimise your cooking time.

3   Spray a large frying pan with low-calorie cooking spray and place over a medium heat. Working in batches of 2–3 fritters, spoon ladlefuls of the mixture into the hot pan and cook for 2–3 minutes until the underside is golden. Flip the fritters and cook on the top-side until golden. Set the cooked fritters aside and repeat until all of your mixture is used up.

TO SERVE

The fritters are now ready to serve with your choice of accompaniments.

TO FREEZE

Set the fritters aside to cool to room temperature, then transfer to a large, labelled freezer bag and freeze flat for up to 3 months.

TO REHEAT FROM FROZEN

These can be defrosted fully in the fridge before reheating or reheated directly from the freezer. If defrosted, place on a foil-lined baking tray and transfer to an oven preheated to 180°C/350°F/gas mark 4 for 8 minutes, until crunchy and golden. If cooking from frozen, cook the same way but increase the cooking time to 12–14 minutes and ensure that the fritters are piping hot all of the way through before serving.

SWEETCORN FRITTERS

PREP: 8–10 MINS **COOK:** 5 MINS **SERVES:** 4 **SUGAR:** 5.8G **KCAL:** 303

Another wonderfully versatile fritter recipe that is sure to be a hit with the whole family. I like a bit of chilli heat in these, but if your family is spice-averse, then simply omit the chilli flakes from the batter. If you are also making the Courgette Fritters (opposite), simply put both pans on the hob side-by-side and cook both types of fritter at the same time. Double bubble!

1½ cups (165g) plain flour
1 tsp baking powder
3 eggs, beaten
3 tbsp low-fat crème fraîche
1 x 165g can sweetcorn, drained
5 spring onions, finely sliced
½ tsp paprika
½ tsp chilli flakes (optional)
½ cup (120ml) milk
low-calorie cooking spray
salt and freshly ground pepper

To serve

Lighter Serve: Low-fat sour cream, sliced avocado and sriracha sauce
Family Serve: Sour cream, guacamole, grated cheese and sriracha

1 Put the flour, baking powder, eggs, crème fraîche, sweetcorn, spring onions, paprika, chilli flakes, milk and a generous grinding of salt and pepper into a large mixing bowl and stir to combine.
2 Spray a large frying pan with low-calorie cooking spray and place over a medium heat. Working in batches of 2–3 fritters, spoon ladlefuls of the mixture into the hot pan and cook for 2–3 minutes until the underside is golden. Flip the fritters and cook on the top-side until golden. Set the cooked fritters aside and repeat until all of your mixture is used up.

TO SERVE

The fritters are now ready to serve with your choice of accompaniments.

TO FREEZE

Set the fritters aside to cool to room temperature, then transfer to a large, labelled freezer bag and freeze flat for up to 3 months.

TO REHEAT FROM FROZEN

These can be defrosted fully in the fridge before reheating or reheated directly from the freezer. If defrosted, place on a foil-lined baking tray and transfer to an oven preheated to 180°C/350°F/gas mark 4 for 8 minutes, until crunchy and golden. If cooking from frozen, cook the same way but increase the cooking time to 12–14 minutes and ensure that the fritters are piping hot all of the way through before serving.

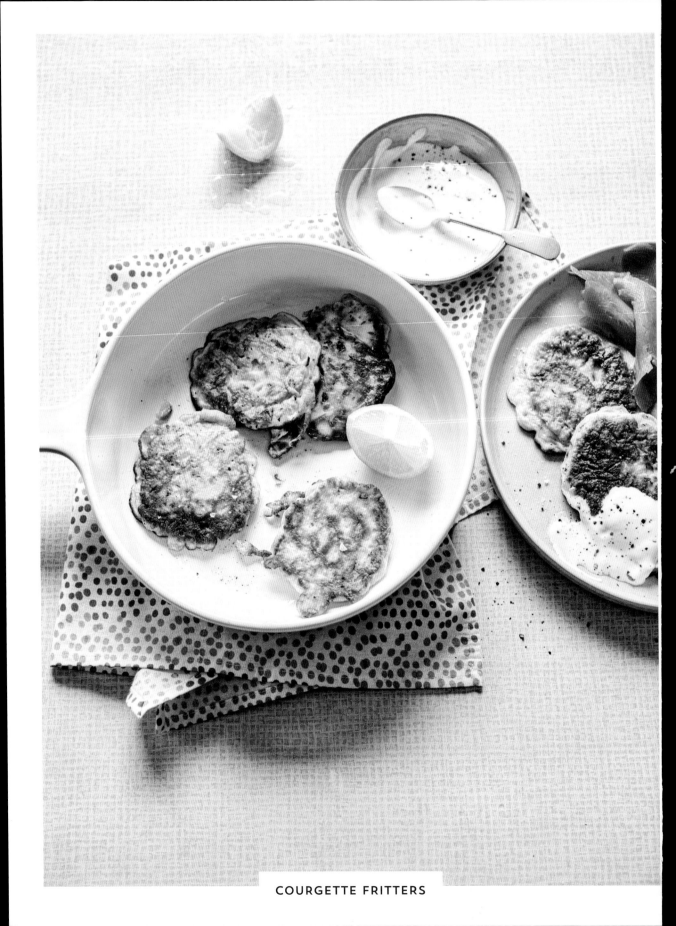

COURGETTE FRITTERS

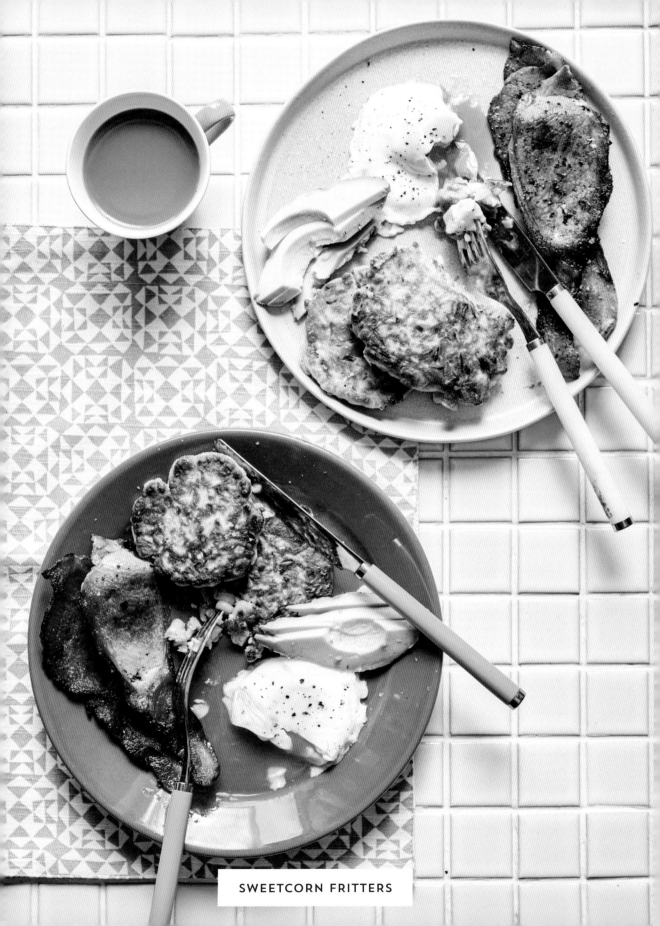

SWEETCORN FRITTERS

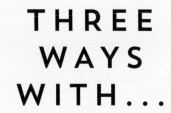

THREE WAYS WITH...

SWEETCORN FRITTERS

Now that you've prepared your Sweetcorn Fritters, what are you going to do with them? Here are three simple ideas for different ways of serving them that will keep mealtimes feeling fresh and different every time. Each meal serves 4.

SWEETCORN FRITTERS WITH CRISPY BACON & FRIED EGGS

1 x quantity Sweetcorn Fritters
   (p.63)
8 rashers bacon (use quorn rashers
   if you are vegetarian)
low-calorie cooking spray
4 eggs

1 Preheat the oven to 180°C/350°F/gas mark 4 and line a baking tray with foil.

2 Cook the Sweetcorn Fritters as per the instructions on page 63.

3 While you are cooking the fritters, lay the bacon on the baking tray and transfer to the oven for around 8 minutes, until crisp.

4 When the fritters and bacon are almost cooked, spray a frying pan with low-calorie cooking spray and place over a medium heat. Once hot, crack the eggs into the pan and fry for 2–3 minutes, until the whites are cooked but the yolks are still runny.

5 Divide the sweetcorn fritters between 4 plates, add a fried egg to each and top with 2 rashers of bacon.

SWEETCORN FRITTERS WITH AVOCADO, CRÈME FRAÎCHE, SRIRACHA & CORIANDER

1 x quantity Sweetcorn Fritters
  (p.63)
2 avocados, stoned, peeled and
  sliced
4 tbsp reduced-fat crème fraîche
sriracha sauce, to taste
1 handful fresh coriander, finely
  chopped

1 Cook the Sweetcorn Fritters as per the instructions on page 63.
2 Once cooked, divide the fritters between 4 plates. Top each with some sliced avocado, a tablespoon of crème fraîche and a drizzle of sriracha sauce. Scatter over the fresh coriander and serve.

SWEETCORN FRITTERS WITH POACHED EGGS & TOMATO RELISH

1 x quantity Sweetcorn Fritters
  (p.63)
4 eggs
4 tbsp shop-bought tomato relish

1 Cook the Sweetcorn Fritters as per the instructions on page 63.
2 Meanwhile, bring a large pan of water to the boil, then reduce to a simmer. Carefully crack 2 of the eggs into the water and leave to cook for 4 minutes, until the white is firm but the yolk is still runny. Remove from the pan with a slotted spoon and repeat with the remaining 2 eggs.
3 Divide the fritters between 4 serving plates and top each plate with a poached egg and a tablespoon of tomato relish. Serve.

MOREISH MINESTRONE

PREP: 5 MINS **COOK:** 40-50 MINS **SERVES:** 4-6 **SUGAR:** 16G **KCAL:** 266

low-calorie cooking spray

1 cup (115g) frozen chopped onions

2 medium carrots, peeled and
finely chopped

2 tsp frozen chopped garlic

2 celery sticks, finely chopped

2 x 400g cans chopped tomatoes

2 tbsp tomato purée

1 tsp dried mixed herbs

3½ cups (840ml) low-sodium
vegetable stock

½ cup (60g) dried macaroni

½ cup (95g) canned red kidney
beans, drained

salt and freshly ground pepper

pre-grated Parmesan cheese,
to serve

To serve

Lighter Serve: Wholemeal pitta
breads

Family Serve: Buttered sourdough
or crusty rolls

> If you are making both soups together, lay out the piles of separate ingredients on the kitchen counter now, then cook the recipes side-by-side as you work.

1 Spray a large saucepan with low-calorie cooking spray and place over a medium heat. Add the onions, carrots, garlic and celery and cook, stirring continuously, for 2–3 minutes, until softened.

2 Add the chopped tomatoes, tomato purée, mixed herbs and stock, then season to taste with salt and pepper. Bring to the boil, then reduce the heat to a gentle simmer and cook, stirring occasionally, for 30–40 minutes, until the vegetables are tender.

> If you are also making the Moroccan Vegetable & Chorizo Soup and you haven't already started it, do so now while this soup is cooking.

TO COOK

Add the macaroni and kidney beans to the pan and continue to cook, stirring occasionally, for 10 minutes, until the pasta is tender. Season the soup to taste, then ladle into bowls, sprinkle with a little grated Parmesan and serve hot.

TO FREEZE

Remove the pan from the heat and set aside until cooled to room temperature. Don't worry that you haven't used the macaroni or kidney beans yet – these will be added on the day of serving. Transfer the soup to a large, labelled freezer bag (a zip-lock bag works best for this) and freeze flat for up to 3 months.

TO COOK FROM FROZEN

Remove the soup from the freezer and leave to defrost fully in the fridge, ideally overnight. Once defrosted, tip the soup into a large saucepan and place over a medium heat. Cook, stirring occasionally, until piping hot all the way through, about 10 minutes, then add the macaroni and kidney beans and continue to cook for another 10 minutes, until the pasta is tender. Season the soup to taste, then ladle into bowls, sprinkle with a little grated Parmesan and serve hot.

MOROCCAN VEGETABLE & CHORIZO SOUP

PREP: 5 MINS **COOK:** 40–50 MINS **SERVES:** 4–6 **SUGAR:** 12G **KCAL:** 242

low-calorie cooking spray
1 cup (115g) frozen chopped
  onions
1 tsp frozen chopped garlic
½ cup (50g) ready-diced chorizo
2 sticks celery, finely chopped
1 tsp ground cumin
1 tbsp tomato purée
2 x 400g cans chopped tomatoes
3½ cups (840ml) low-sodium
  chicken or vegetable stock
1 x 400g can chickpeas, drained
salt and freshly ground pepper

To serve
Lighter Serve: Wholemeal pitta
breads
Family Serve: Buttered sourdough
or crusty rolls

1 Spray a large saucepan with low-calorie cooking spray and place over a medium heat. Add the onions, garlic and chorizo and cook, stirring continuously, for 2–3 minutes, until the vegetables have softened and the chorizo has started to release its oil.
2 Add the celery, cumin, tomato purée, chopped tomatoes and stock and stir to combine. Bring to the boil, then reduce the heat to a gentle simmer and cook, stirring occasionally, for 30–40 minutes, until the vegetables are tender.
3 Add the chickpeas to the soup and continue to cook, stirring occasionally, for another 10 minutes.

TO SERVE

Season the soup to taste, then ladle into bowls and serve hot.

TO FREEZE

Remove the pan from the heat and set aside until cooled to room temperature. Transfer the soup to a large, labelled freezer bag (a zip-lock bag works best for this) and freeze flat for up to 3 months.

TO REHEAT FROM FROZEN

This can be defrosted in the fridge overnight and then reheated in a pan until piping hot, or cooked from frozen. If cooking from frozen, tip the frozen soup into a large pan, cover with a lid and place over a low heat. Cook the soup, removing the lid occasionally and breaking it up with a wooden spoon as the mixture defrosts, until fully defrosted and piping hot all of the way through.

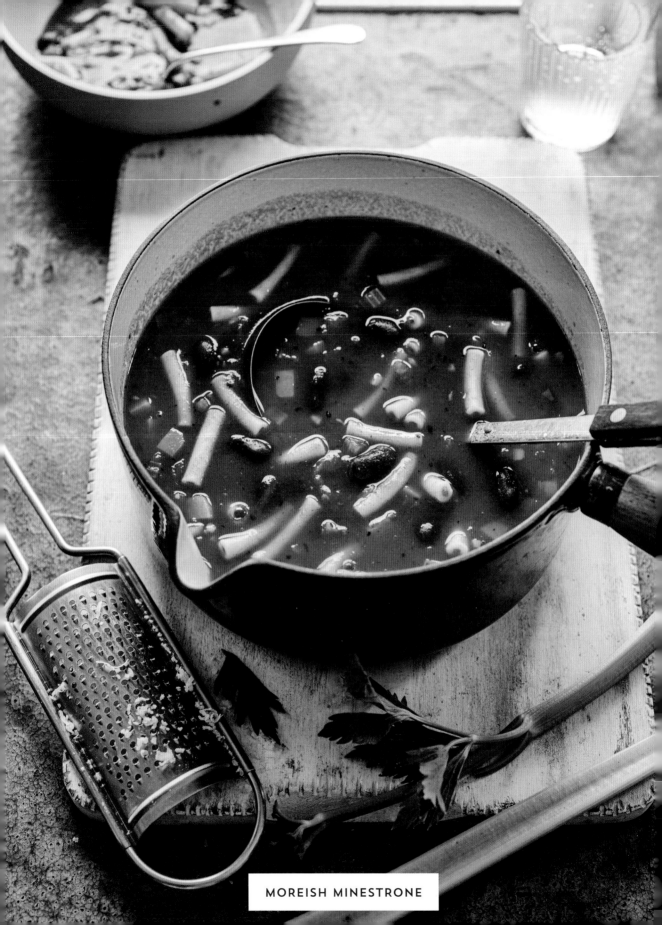

MOREISH MINESTRONE

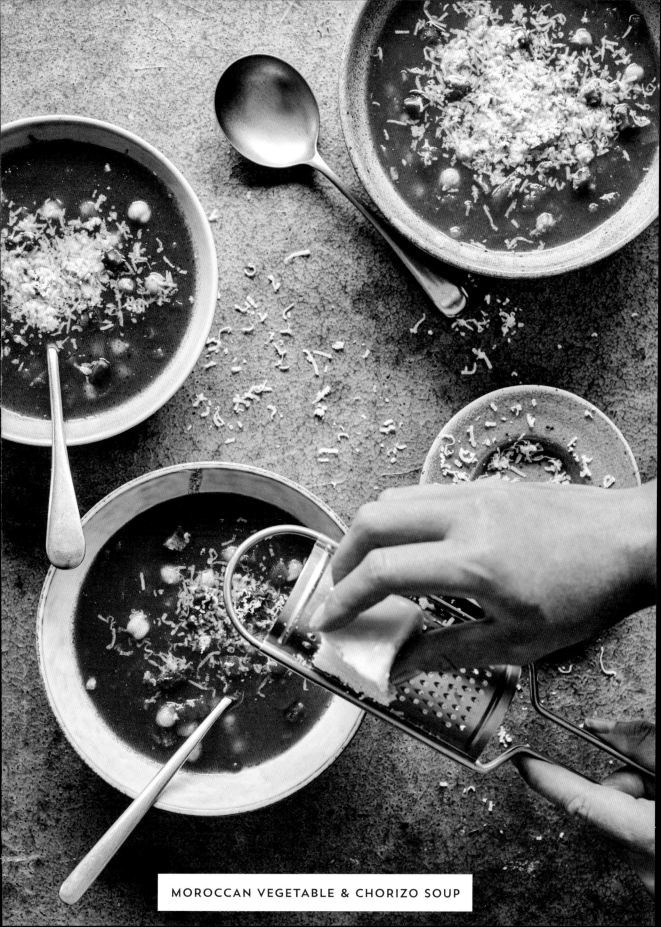

MOROCCAN VEGETABLE & CHORIZO SOUP

KEDGEREE

PREP: 10 MINS **COOK:** 10 MINS **SERVES:** 4 **SUGAR:** 10G **KCAL:** 419

1 cup (190g) basmati rice

3 eggs

1½ cups (360ml) semi-skimmed milk

2 fresh skinless smoked haddock fillets

1 tbsp low-fat margarine

1 cup (115g) frozen chopped onions

2 cups (310g) frozen peas

1 tsp mild curry powder

salt and freshly ground pepper

small bunch parsley, leaves chopped, to serve

1 Add the rice and eggs, still in their shells, to a large saucepan and pour over boiling water to cover. Place the pan over a medium heat and bring to the boil, then reduce the heat to a gentle simmer and leave to cook for 10 minutes.

2 Meanwhile, bring the milk to a simmer over a low heat in a frying pan, then add the haddock fillets and cook for around 8 minutes, until flaky.

> If you are also making the frittata, pan-fry the salmon now while the rice and fish for the kedgeree are cooking.

3 Flake the cooked fish into a bowl and set aside. Remove the frying pan from the heat and decant the milk into a small jug. Set aside for later.

4 If you are making this ahead to freeze, remove the eggs from the pan, and drain and rinse the rice at the end of the 10-minute cooking time. If you are making this to eat now, remove the eggs from the pan but continue cooking the rice until it is tender before draining and rinsing. Peel and quarter the eggs and set both the rice and eggs aside for later.

5 Using the same pan that you cooked the fish in, melt the margarine over a medium heat, then add the onions, peas and curry powder and cook, stirring continuously, for 2–3 minutes, until the onions are soft.

6 Tip the rice and fish into the frying pan and stir to combine with the spiced onion and pea mixture. Add 2 tablespoons of the reserved milk and a generous grinding of salt and pepper, and stir again.

7 Arrange the quartered eggs over the top of the kedgeree.

TO COOK

Scatter the kedgeree with freshly chopped parsley and place in the middle of the table for everyone to dig in.

TO FREEZE

Leave the kedgeree aside to cool to room temperature, then transfer to a large, labelled freezer bag and freeze flat for up to 3 months.

TO REHEAT FROM FROZEN

This can be defrosted overnight in the fridge or reheated straight from frozen. If defrosted, transfer the kedgeree to a large, microwaveable bowl and cook on high for 6–8 minutes, until piping hot all of the way through. If reheating from frozen, use the defrost setting on your microwave and ensure the dish is piping hot all of the way through before serving. Scatter over freshly chopped parsley to serve.

SALMON, PEA & LEEK FRITTATA

PREP: 5 MINS **COOK:** 20–25 MINS **SERVES:** 4 **SUGAR:** 4.4G **KCAL:** 362

This frittata is filled with all the good things and can easily be adapted to whatever vegetables you have to hand. It is great for lunches or grab-and-go dinners as, once frozen, individual slices can quickly be defrosted.

low-calorie cooking spray
2 fresh salmon fillets, skin-on
1 cup (115g) frozen peas
1 cup (150g) frozen sliced leeks or
   1 medium leek, finely sliced
1 cup (115g) frozen chopped
   onions
8 eggs
1 tsp dried dill
salt and freshly ground pepper

To serve
Lighter Serve: Green salad and
your choice of dressing (p.210–11)
Family Serve: Buttered new
potatoes, salad and your choice of
dressing (p.210–11)

1 Preheat the oven to 180°C/350°F/gas mark 4. Spray a round, 20cm (8in) baking dish with low-calorie cooking spray and line with baking parchment.

2 Spray a frying pan with low-calorie cooking spray and place over a medium heat. Once hot, add the salmon fillets to the pan, skin-side down, and cook for 5 minutes, then flip over and cook for another 5 minutes on the top-side, until the salmon is cooked through.

3 Transfer the salmon to a board and remove and discard the skin. Flake the salmon flesh and scatter over the base of the prepared baking dish.

4 Return the frying pan to the heat, adding more low-calorie cooking spray, if necessary, and add the peas, leeks and onions. Cook, stirring continuously, for 3–4 minutes until softened. Tip the pea and onion mixture into the baking dish with the salmon and spread everything out in an even layer.

5 Crack the eggs into a mixing bowl and add the dried dill and a generous grinding of salt and pepper. Beat the egg mixture until well combined, then pour over the fish and vegetable mixture in the baking dish. Using a fork, check to ensure that all of the filling ingredients are distributed evenly throughout the egg mixture.

6 Transfer the baking dish to the oven and cook for 20–25 minutes, until the frittata is just cooked through.

TO SERVE

Leave the frittata in the dish for 5 minutes to firm-up and cool slightly, then carefully slide out of the dish and onto a large chopping board. Slice the frittata and serve warm with your choice of accompaniments.

TO FREEZE

Leave the frittata in the dish to cool to room temperature, then carefully slide out and onto a large chopping board. Slice the frittata into wedges and transfer to a large, labelled freezer bag. Freeze flat for up to 3 months.

TO REHEAT FROM FROZEN

The frittata can be defrosted in the fridge first or reheated directly from frozen. If defrosted, simply reheat the slices in the microwave until piping hot all the way through. If reheating from frozen, wrap the slices in foil and transfer to an oven preheated to 180°C/350°F/gas mark 4 for 20–25 minutes until piping hot all of the way through.

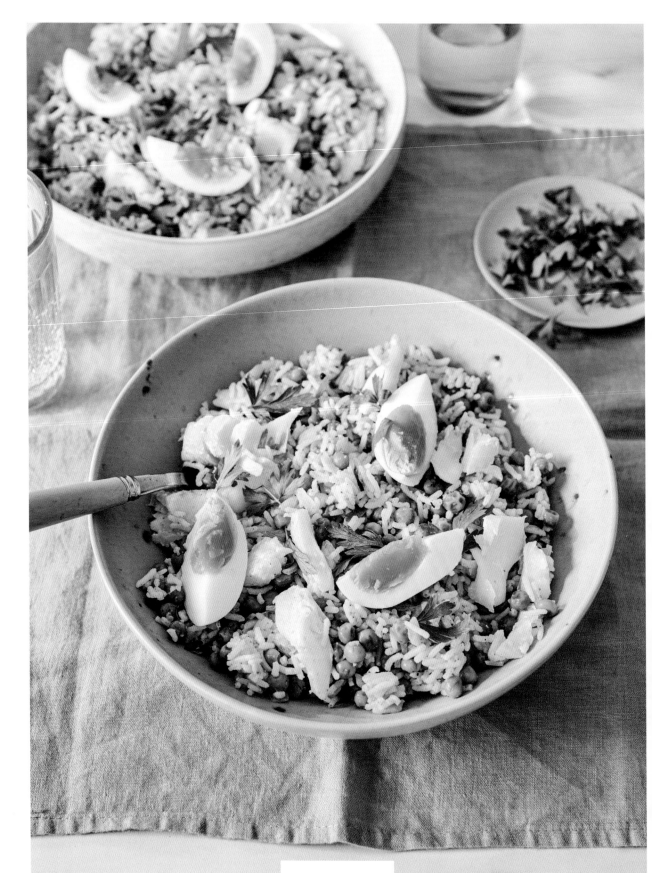

KEDGEREE

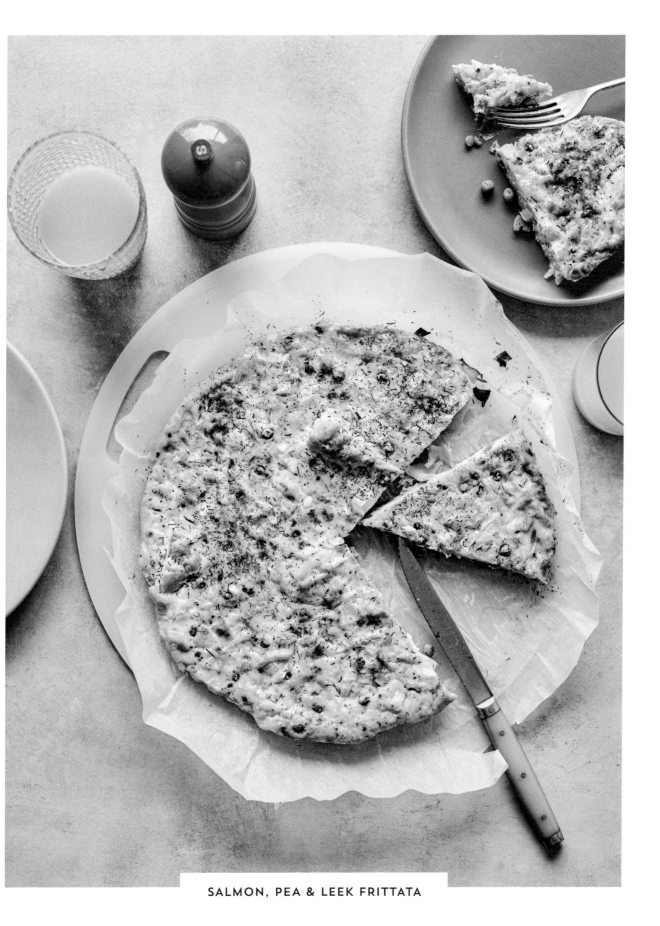

SALMON, PEA & LEEK FRITTATA

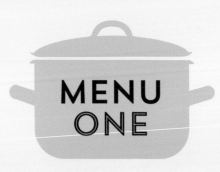

3 FOR THE FRIDGE,
3 FOR THE FREEZER

Are you ready to batch three family meals for the week ahead and three to store in the freezer for another time in just 45 minutes? You will be making three recipes, each of which is doubled-up to feed eight people, so you simply need to split the recipe into two family meals before freezing one and putting the other in the fridge for the week ahead. The recipes are a mixture of cooked and no-cook freezer-bag meals, so while one recipe is bubbling away on the stove or cooking in the oven, you can be making the next meal ready for the fridge and freezer.

The shopping list on the opposite page includes everything you need and I have scaled up the ingredients for you so you don't need to worry about doubling the recipe. Simply buy what's on the shopping list and you will have everything you need to make the six meals. Once you have your shopping, lay the ingredients out into piles according to the groupings overleaf, so you have exactly what you need for each recipe to hand. Then simply follow the numbered guide and you can't go wrong!

Don't panic if this takes you more than 45 minutes the first time you cook it – you will get quicker each time you make it. So, roll up your sleeves, get cooking and think about the time you will be saving yourself in the future!

YOU WILL BE MAKING:

VEGETABLE & VEGGIE SAUSAGE ONE-PAN BAKE ⓥ
BUTTERNUT SQUASH & COCONUT SOUP ⓥ
SUMMERY COUSCOUS SALAD ⓥ

SHOPPING LIST

Fresh

2 x 300g packs pre-diced butternut
squash and sweet potato mix

8 red peppers

4 yellow peppers

4 red onions

8 medium-sized sweet potatoes

4 lemons

2 x 200g packs low-fat feta cheese

Frozen

1 x 500g bag frozen chopped onions

1 x 75g bag frozen chopped garlic

1 x 75g bag frozen chopped ginger

1 x 50g pack frozen chopped coriander

16 frozen vegetarian sausages

Storecupboard

low-calorie cooking spray

olive oil

2 x 400g cans reduced-fat coconut milk

4 tsp paprika

2 tsp chilli flakes (optional)

1 x 500g pack dried couscous

4 low-sodium vegetable stock cubes

salt and pepper

INGREDIENTS

BUTTERNUT SQUASH & COCONUT SOUP

low-calorie cooking spray
2 cups (230g) frozen chopped onions
2 tsp frozen chopped garlic
4 tsp frozen chopped ginger
2 x 300g packs pre-diced butternut squash and sweet potato mix
4 red peppers, deseeded and diced
4 cups (960ml) low-sodium vegetable stock
2 tsp frozen chopped coriander
2 x 400g cans reduced-fat coconut milk

SUMMERY COUSCOUS SALAD

2 cups (360g) dried couscous
2 cups (480ml) low-sodium vegetable stock
2 red onions, finely chopped
2 red peppers, deseeded and diced
2 yellow peppers, deseeded and diced
2 small sweet potatoes, peeled and chopped into 2.5cm (1in) cubes
6 tbsp olive oil
juice of 4 lemons
2 x 200g packs low-fat feta cheese
salt and freshly ground pepper

VEGETABLE & VEGGIE SAUSAGE ONE-PAN BAKE

2 red onions, cut into wedges
2 yellow peppers, deseeded and cut into 2.5cm (1in) pieces
2 red peppers, deseeded and cut into 2.5cm (1in) pieces
6 medium sweet potatoes, peeled and chopped into 2.5cm (1in) cubes
4 tsp frozen chopped garlic
4 tsp paprika
2 tsp chilli flakes (optional)
4 tbsp olive oil
16 frozen vegetarian sausages
salt and freshly ground pepper

METHOD

1 Preheat the oven to 180°C/350°F/gas mark 4.

BUTTERNUT SQUASH & COCONUT SOUP

2 Spray a large saucepan with low-calorie cooking spray and place over a medium heat. Add the onions, garlic and ginger and cook, stirring continuously, for 2–3 minutes, until softened.

3 Add the butternut squash and sweet potato mix, red peppers, vegetable stock and coriander to the pan and stir to combine. Bring to the boil, then reduce the heat to a simmer and leave to cook for 15 minutes, stirring occasionally.

SUMMERY COUSCOUS SALAD

4 Put the couscous in a large bowl and pour over the vegetable stock. Stir once, cover with a tea towel and set aside for 10 minutes.

5 Put the chopped red onions, red and yellow peppers and sweet potatoes on a foil-lined baking tray and drizzle with 2 tablespoons of the olive oil. Season with a generous grinding of salt and pepper and transfer to the preheated oven for 20 minutes, until the veg are tender.

BUTTERNUT SQUASH & COCONUT SOUP CONTINUED…

6 Return to the soup and add the 2 cans of coconut milk to the pan and stir to combine. Bring back to the boil, then reduce the heat to a simmer and leave to cook for a further 15 minutes, until all the vegetables are tender.

VEGETABLE & VEGGIE SAUSAGE ONE-PAN BAKE

7 Set 2 large, labelled freezer bags side-by-side on the counter. Into each bag add half of the prepared onions, peppers and sweet potatoes. Next add 2 teaspoons of garlic, 2 teaspoons of paprika, 1 teaspoon of chilli flakes, if using, 2 tablespoons of olive oil and a generous grinding of salt and pepper to each bag. Massage the bags gently to ensure the veg are coated in the oil and spices.

8 Divide the sausages equally between 2 smaller freezer bags, seal and place 1 bag in each of the larger bags with the vegetables. Seal the larger bags. Transfer 1 of the bags to the freezer and freeze flat for up to 3 months, transfer the other bag to the fridge to use in the coming week.

CONTINUED OVERLEAF…

BUTTERNUT SQUASH & COCONUT SOUP CONTINUED...

9 The vegetables should now be tender. Remove the soup from the heat and set aside to cool while you complete the couscous salad.

SUMMERY COUSCOUS SALAD CONTINUED...

10 Fluff the couscous up with a fork and set aside.

11 Once cooked, remove the vegetables from the oven and set aside to cool for 10 minutes. (This is a good time to wipe down your surfaces, doing any washing up and get organised with freezer bags or soup containers for storing your completed meals.)

12 Once cooled, tip the vegetables into the couscous along with the remaining 4 tablespoons of olive oil, the lemon juice, crumbled feta cheese and a generous grinding of salt and pepper. Give everything a good mix to combine.

13 Put half of the mixture into a large, labelled freezer bag and freeze flat for up to 3 months. Put the remaining half in another bag or plastic container with a lid and store in the fridge for the week ahead.

BUTTERNUT SQUASH & COCONUT SOUP CONTINUED...

14 Blend the cooled soup until smooth with a handheld stick blender. Put half of the mixture into a large, labelled freezer bag (a zip-lock bag works best for this) and freeze flat for up to 3 months.

Put the remaining half in another bag or plastic container with a lid and store in the fridge for the week ahead.

Congratulations!

You have just made six meals!
Three for the week ahead
and three for the freezer.

WHEN YOU COME TO COOK

Once cooked, all of these meals are best fully defrosted before cooking. All reheated meals should reach a temperature of 74°C/165°F. Always make sure any reheated food is piping hot before serving. Cooking instructions for each dish are given below.

BUTTERNUT SQUASH & COCONUT SOUP

FROM THE FRIDGE

Pour the soup into a large pan and place over a medium heat until piping hot.

FROM THE FREEZER

Remove the soup from the freezer and leave to fully defrost in the fridge, ideally overnight. Once defrosted, pour the soup into a large pan and place over a medium heat until piping hot.

To serve
Lighter Serve: Wholemeal pitta breads
Family Serve: Cooked noodles added and Light-And-Easy Naan Breads (p.208) alongside.

SUMMERY COUSCOUS SALAD

FROM THE FRIDGE

The salad is ready to serve. Simply tip into a serving bowl and enjoy.

FROM THE FREEZER

Remove the salad from the freezer and leave to defrost at room temperature. This should only take about 2 hours. Once defrosted, the salad is ready to serve. If it has dried out in the freezer, drizzle with a little extra olive oil.

To serve
Lighter Serve: A large, leafy salad
Family Serve: Salad, hummus and pitta breads

VEGETABLE & VEGGIE SAUSAGE ONE-PAN BAKE

FROM THE FRIDGE

Preheat the oven to 180°C/350°F/gas mark 4. Tip the vegetable mixture into a roasting tin and transfer to the oven for 20 minutes. After 20 minutes, toss the vegetables and add the sausages. Return to the oven for another 20 minutes, until the vegetables are tender and the sausages are golden and cooked through.

FROM THE FREEZER

Remove the sausage-and-vegetable bag from the freezer and leave to fully defrost in the fridge, ideally overnight. Once defrosted, cook as directed in the *From the Fridge* section, above.

FAKEAWAYS

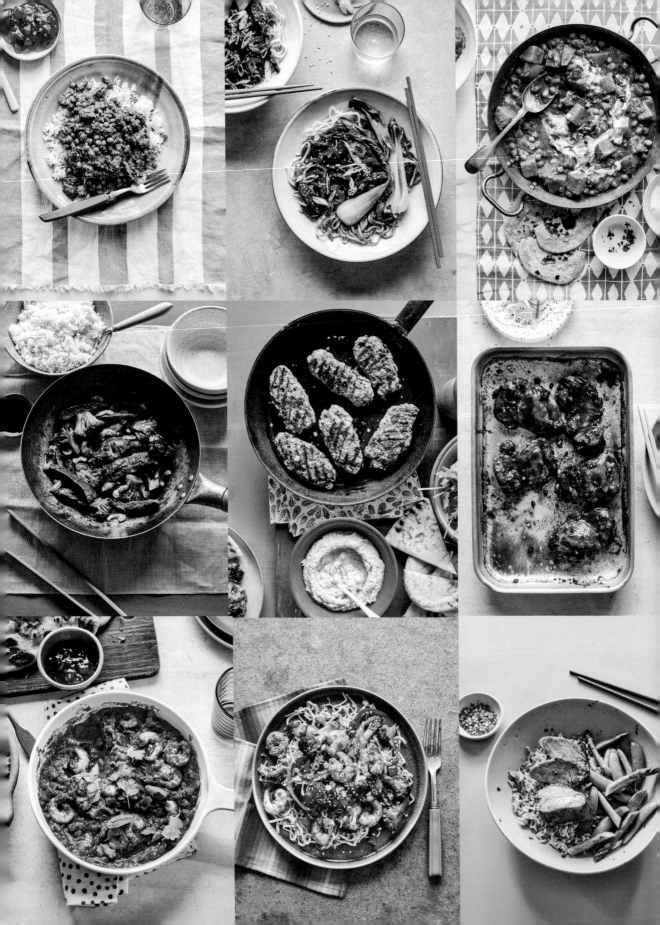

FAKEAWAYS

A Friday-night curry or Chinese takeaway delivered straight to your door is a wonderful thing, but in the interests of healthy eating, is best left as an occasional treat. The good news is that you can emulate the flavours of your favourite takeaway dishes at home, but with much lighter end results. In this chapter, you'll find my takes on these dishes, but with simple subs and low-calorie serving suggestions, to make them just that little bit healthier.

For kebab lovers, my Lamb Koftas (p.90) or Greek Lemon & Herb Chicken (p.91) are delicious served in salad-packed pitta breads with hummus or harissa dressing on the side, and can be transformed into something more substantial by adding the Skin-On Chips (p.204) or Piri-Piri Sweet Potato Chips (p.205) from the sides section of this book. For lovers of Asian food, my Sticky Asian Beef (p.86) and Soy Beef & Broccoli (p.87) are both packed with flavour and wonderfully light. Low-sodium soy sauce is readily available and really helps keep the salt down in these dishes, so is worth seeking out. For vegetarians, my fragrant Chickpea & Sweet Potato Curry (p.100) is always a treat and is packed full of healthy veg.

The *3 for the Fridge, 3 for the Freezer* section (p.108–113) in this chapter has three quick, easy and healthy takes on takeaway classics. Fill your fridge and freezer with Sweet & Sour Chicken, Kung Pao Pork and Thai Sea Bass Parcels and you'll never need to scrabble around for that takeaway menu again.

STICKY ASIAN BEEF

PREP: 5 MINS **COOK:** 8 MINS **SERVES:** 4 **SUGAR:** 5.7G **KCAL:** 283

This quick stir-fried beef dish is full of flavour and can easily be paired with stir-fried veg and noodles or rice for a more substantial meal. I always double this recipe and freeze one for another day, as the most time-consuming part is taking the ingredients out of the cupboard!

4 tbsp low-sodium soy sauce
2 tbsp hoisin sauce
2 tsp frozen chopped garlic
2 tsp frozen chopped ginger
1 tbsp white wine vinegar
2 tsp cornflour
4 spring onions, sliced
1 tsp frozen chopped chilli
  (optional)
1 tbsp sesame oil
600g beef stir-fry strips
sesame seeds, to serve

To serve
Lighter Serve: Cauliflower Rice
(p.203) and tenderstem broccoli
Family Serve: On a bed of
wholewheat noodles with
tenderstem broccoli

1 Put the soy sauce, hoisin sauce, garlic, ginger, white wine vinegar, cornflour, spring onions and chilli, if using, into a small bowl and mix well to combine.

TO COOK

Heat the sesame oil in a wok or large frying pan over a medium-high heat. Add the beef and cook, stirring continuously, for 4–6 minutes, until the beef is almost cooked to your liking. Add the sauce and stir to coat the beef. If you would like a saucy (rather than sticky) end dish, also add ½ cup (120ml) of boiling water. Serve hot with your choice of accompaniments and with the sesame seeds scattered over the top.

TO FREEZE

Transfer the uncooked beef strips to a large, labelled freezer bag, but do not seal. Transfer the sauce to a smaller freezer bag and seal, then place this bag into the larger bag with the beef. Seal the larger bag and freeze flat for up to 3 months.

TO COOK FROM FROZEN

Remove the bag containing the beef and the sauce from the freezer and leave to defrost fully in the fridge, ideally overnight. Once defrosted, cook and serve the beef as described in the *To Cook* section, left.

SOY BEEF & BROCCOLI

PREP: 5 MINS **COOK:** 10 MINS **SERVES:** 4 **SUGAR:** 9.5G **KCAL:** 285

This stir-fried beef recipe contains many similar ingredients to the Sticky Asian Beef (opposite), so it is easy to bag both up for the freezer at the same time.

4 tbsp low-sodium soy sauce
2 tbsp Sweet Chilli Sauce (p.215 or store-bought)
1 tsp frozen chopped garlic
2 tsp frozen chopped ginger
1 tsp cornflour
1 tbsp sesame oil
400g beef stir-fry strips
2 cups (350g) frozen broccoli florets
2 handfuls unsalted cashew nuts

To serve

Lighter Serve: Cauliflower Rice (p.203) and stir-fried pak choi
Family Serve: On a bed of wholewheat noodles with stir-fried pak choi

1 Put the soy sauce, sweet chilli sauce, garlic, ginger and cornflour into a small bowl and mix well to combine.

TO COOK

Heat the sesame oil in a wok or frying pan over a medium-high heat. Add the beef and cook, stirring, for 2 minutes. Add the broccoli and continue to cook for 3–4 minutes, until the beef is almost cooked to your liking. Add the sauce to the pan along with the cashews and stir to coat the beef. If you would like a saucy (rather than sticky) end dish, also add ½ cup (120ml) of boiling water. Serve hot.

TO FREEZE

Transfer the uncooked beef strips to a large, labelled freezer bag, but do not seal. Transfer the sauce to a smaller freezer bag and seal, then place this bag into the larger bag with the beef. Seal the larger bag and freeze flat for up to 3 months.

TO COOK FROM FROZEN

Remove the bag containing the beef and the sauce from the freezer and leave to defrost fully in the fridge, ideally overnight. Once defrosted, cook and serve the beef as described in the *To Cook* section, left.

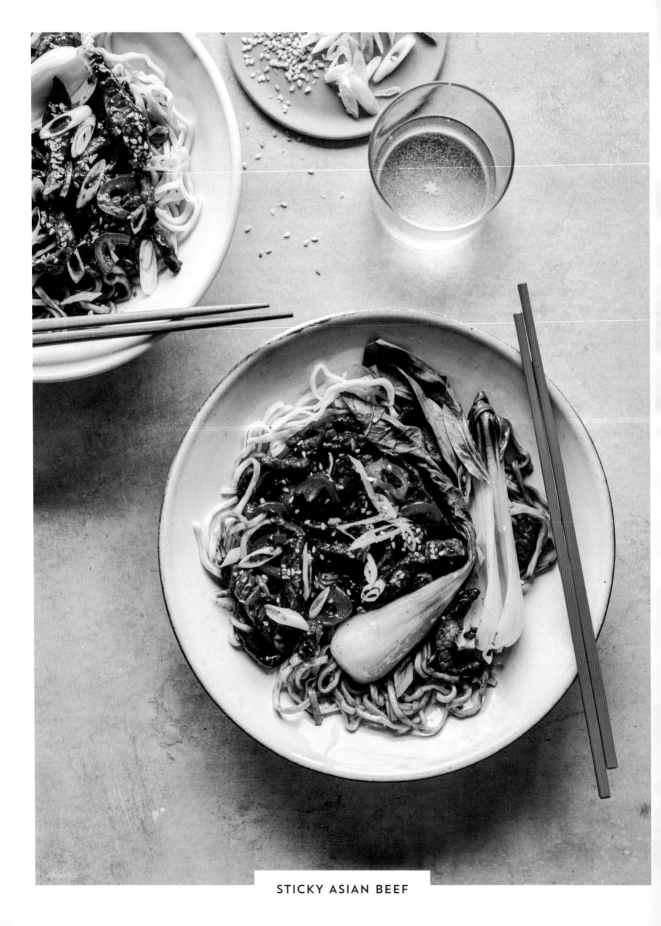

STICKY ASIAN BEEF

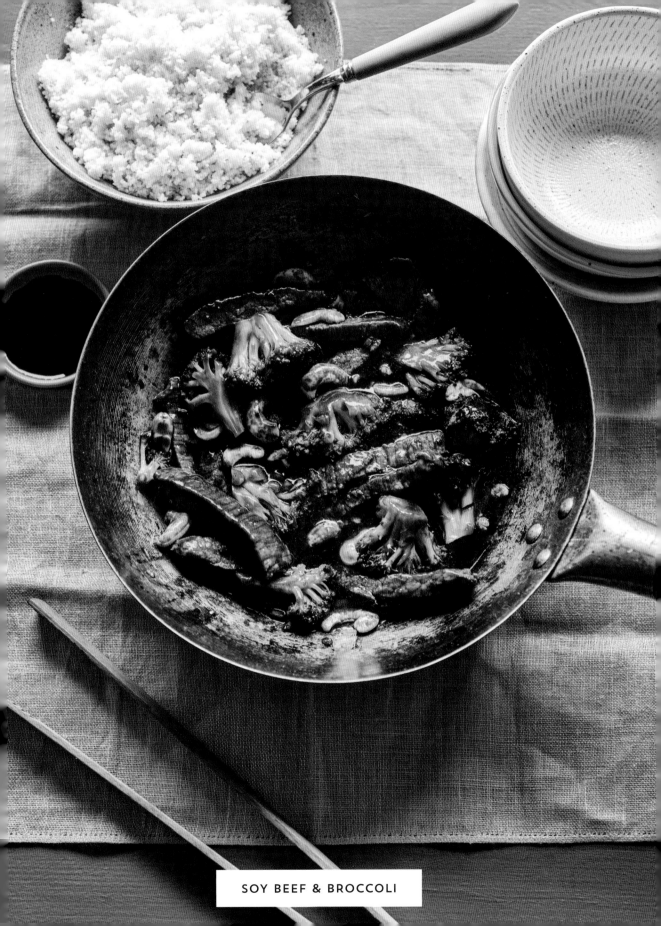

SOY BEEF & BROCCOLI

LAMB KOFTAS

PREP: 10 MINS **COOK:** 8 MINS **SERVES:** 4 **SUGAR:** 0G **KCAL:** 254

These flavour-packed lamb koftas are brilliant served in a pitta bread for a light meal, or with chips or wedges for a more substantial meal. They can be cooked directly from the freezer, so are great to have on hand for those days when you've forgotten to get something out to defrost the evening before.

500g lean lamb mince
2 tsp frozen chopped garlic
2 tsp ground cumin
1 tsp ground coriander
1 tsp frozen chopped parsley
1 tsp dried mint
low-calorie cooking spray
salt and freshly ground pepper

To serve
Lighter Serve: Wholemeal pitta breads with salad and hummus
Family Serve: Skin-On Chips (p.204), salad and hummus

1 Put the lamb, garlic, cumin, coriander, parsley and mint in a large mixing bowl and season with a generous grinding of salt and pepper.
2 Using your hands, bring all of the ingredients together until well combined, then divide the mixture into 8 equal-sized balls. You can leave the koftas as ball shapes or squeeze them into slightly flattened sausage shapes, depending on your preference.

TO COOK

Spray a griddle or frying pan with low-calorie cooking spray and place over a medium heat. Once hot, add the koftas and cook, turning regularly, for around 8 minutes, until cooked all the way through.

TO FREEZE

Lay the uncooked koftas on a lined baking tray and transfer to the freezer for an hour to allow them to firm up. Transfer the part-frozen koftas to a large, labelled freezer bag and freeze flat for up to 3 months.

TO COOK FROM FROZEN

These can be defrosted overnight in the fridge or cooked straight from the freezer. If defrosted, cook as described in the To Cook section, left. If cooking from frozen, cook the koftas in the same way but increase the cooking time to 16 minutes and place the pan over a low heat at the start of cooking, gradually turning the heat up to medium as the koftas start to cook. Ensure the koftas are piping hot all the way through before serving.

GREEK LEMON & HERB CHICKEN

PREP: 5 MINS **COOK:** 10 MINS **SERVES:** 4 **SUGAR:** 1.3G **KCAL:** 174

This is a great dish to make ahead and store in the freezer to whip out for a quick-win dinner. It's really tasty and versatile and can be served in pittas with hummus and salad as described below, added to salads or, for a treat, with wedges or chips alongside. Easy and delicious.

½ cup (110g) Greek yoghurt
juice of 1 lemon
1 tsp frozen chopped chilli
1 tsp frozen chopped garlic
1 tsp paprika
1 tsp dried oregano
4 skinless, boneless chicken
   breasts, cut into bite-sized
   pieces
low-calorie cooking spray
salt and freshly ground pepper

To serve

Lighter Serve: Pitta breads, shredded iceberg lettuce, sliced tomatoes and hummus
Family Serve: As above, with Skin-On Chips (p.204) on the side

1   Put the yoghurt, lemon juice, chilli, garlic, paprika and oregano into a large bowl, season with salt and pepper and stir to combine.

TO COOK

If you are making this to serve now, add the cut-up chicken to the bowl and stir to combine with the marinade. Cover and set aside in the fridge to marinate for at least 30 minutes. Once marinated, remove the chicken from the marinade and shake off any excess. Spray a frying pan with low-calorie cooking spray, place over a medium heat and fry the chicken for 5–10 minutes, turning occasionally, until cooked through. Serve hot.

TO FREEZE

Place the raw chicken pieces in a large, labelled, freezer bag and pour over the marinade. Massage the bag with your hands to make sure the chicken is well coated, then seal the bag, expelling any air, and freeze flat for up to 3 months.

TO COOK FROM FROZEN

Remove the bag from the freezer and leave to completely defrost in the fridge, ideally overnight. Once defrosted, remove the chicken from the marinade (don't worry if it looks like the marinade has split in the freezer) and cook in a large frying pan over a medium heat for 5–10 minutes, turning occasionally, until cooked through. Serve hot.

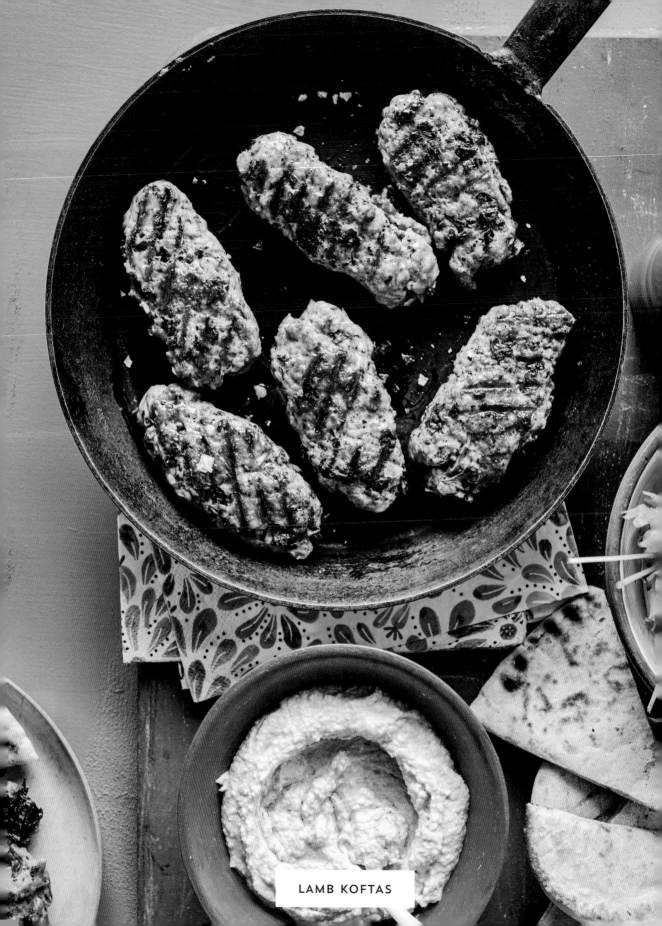

LAMB KOFTAS

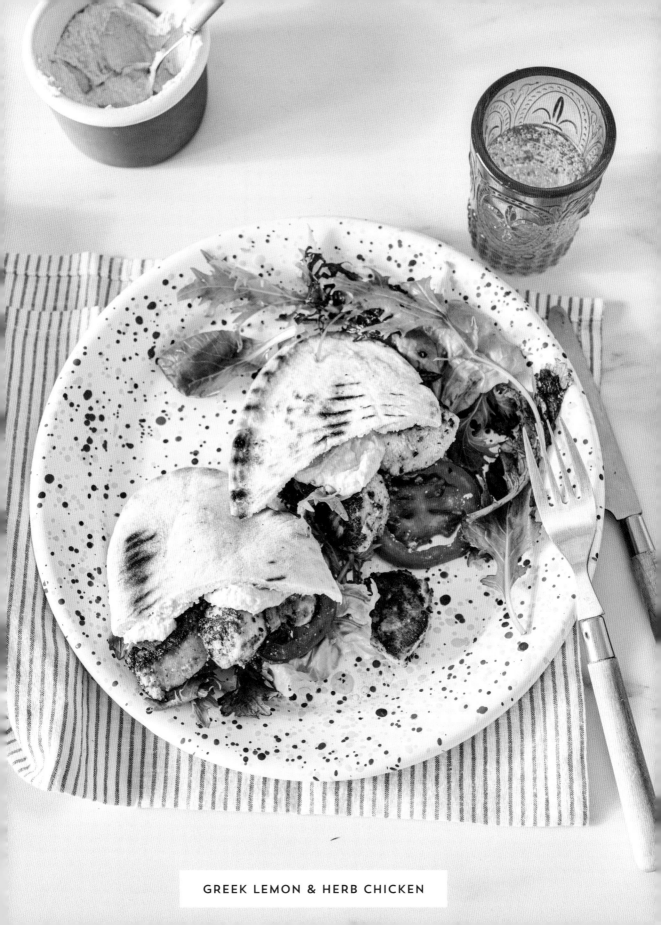

GREEK LEMON & HERB CHICKEN

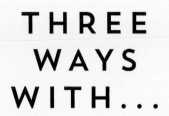

THREE WAYS WITH...

LAMB KOFTAS

Now that you've prepared your Lamb Koftas, what are you going to do with them? Here are three simple ideas for different ways of serving them that will keep mealtimes feeling fresh and different every time. Each meal serves 4.

LAMB KOFTAS WITH PAPRIKA FLATBREADS & HARISSA DRESSING

1 x quantity Lamb Koftas (p.90)
4 Light-And-Easy Paprika
  Flatbreads (p.209)
1 x quantity Harissa Dressing
  (p.210)
1 pack mixed salad leaves
1 handful cherry tomatoes

1 Cook the Lamb Koftas as per the instructions on page 90.
2 Cook the Paprika Flatbreads as per the instructions on page 209.
3 Divide the flatbreads between 4 serving plates and add 2 koftas to each flatbread. Drizzle with the Harissa Dressing and serve with salad leaves and cherry tomatoes on the side.

LAMB KOFTAS WITH SKIN-ON CHIPS & SALAD

1 x quantity Skin-On Chips
  (p.204)
1 x quantity Lamb Koftas (p.90)
1 pack mixed salad leaves
1 handful cherry tomatoes

1   Cook the Skin-On Chips as per the instructions on page 204.
2   While they are cooking, prepare and cook the Lamb Koftas as per the instructions on page 90.
3   Divide the chips and koftas between 4 serving plates and serve with salad leaves and cherry tomatoes on the side.

LAMB KOFTAS WITH COUSCOUS, HUMMUS & SALAD

1½ cups (270g) dried couscous
1 x quantity Lamb Koftas (p.90)
100g low-fat feta cheese,
  crumbled
4 tbsp shop-bought hummus
1 pack mixed salad leaves
salt and freshly ground pepper

1   Put the couscous in a bowl and pour over 2¼ cups (540ml) of boiling water. Stir once, cover with a tea towel and set aside for 10 minutes, while you start making the koftas.
2   Meanwhile, cook the Lamb Koftas as per the instructions on page 90.
3   After 10 minutes, fluff up the couscous with a fork and season to taste with salt and pepper.
4   Divide the couscous between 4 serving plates, top each pile with 2 lamb koftas and scatter over the feta cheese. Serve with the hummus and salad leaves alongside.

PRAWN CURRY

PREP: 5 MINS **COOK:** 30 MINS **SERVES:** 4 **SUGAR:** 13G **KCAL:** 205

Sweet and succulent prawns make a wonderful speedy addition to a curry, as they can be cooked quickly in the curry sauce just before serving. If you are making this ahead for the freezer, simply freeze the curry sauce alongside the prawns and remove them both to defrost at the same time. If you want to make this fresh, do remember that the prawns will need to be defrosted before you start making your curry sauce as they cannot be cooked from frozen.

low calorie cooking spray
1 cup (115g) frozen chopped onions
2 tsp frozen chopped garlic
2 tbsp tikka masala spice paste
1 tsp ground cumin
2 tbsp tomato purée
2 x 400g cans chopped tomatoes
½ cup (120ml) low-sodium
  vegetable stock
300g frozen raw king prawns
  (defrosted on the day you want
  to serve the curry)

To serve
Lighter Serve: Cauliflower Rice (p.203) and a sprinkling of fresh coriander leaves
Family Serve: Basmati rice, Light-And-Easy Naan Breads (p.208) and a spoonful of yoghurt

1   Spray a large saucepan with low-calorie cooking spray and place over a medium heat. Add the onions and garlic and cook, stirring, for 2–3 minutes, until softened.
2   Add the spice paste and cumin and cook for a further minute, then add the tomato purée, chopped tomatoes and vegetable stock and stir to combine. Bring to the boil, then reduce the heat to a gentle simmer and leave to cook, stirring occasionally, for 25 minutes, until the sauce has reduced and thickened.

If you are also making the Prawn Stir-Fry for the freezer, assemble this now while the curry sauce is cooking.

TO COOK

If you are making this to serve straightaway, add the defrosted prawns to the pan with the sauce and leave to cook for 5 minutes more. Prawns can overcook quickly, so keep an eye on them and remove the pan from the heat as soon as they are cooked through. Serve the curry hot with your choice of accompaniments.

TO FREEZE

Remove the pan from the heat and set aside to cool to room temperature. Once cool, transfer the curry sauce to a large, labelled freezer bag (a zip-lock bag works best for this) and freeze flat for up to 3 months. I like to freeze the curry sauce next to the frozen prawns so that they can easily be removed from the freezer and defrosted at the same time.

TO COOK FROM FROZEN

Remove the frozen prawns and curry sauce from the freezer and leave to defrost in the fridge, ideally overnight. Once defrosted, pour the curry sauce into a large saucepan and cook, stirring occasionally, over a low heat until piping hot. Add the prawns and continue to cook for 5 minutes more. Serve hot.

PRAWN STIR-FRY

PREP: 5 MINS **COOK:** 10 MINS **SERVES:** 4 **SUGAR:** 13G **KCAL:** 222

1 tbsp sesame oil

1 head broccoli, cut into small florets

1 cup (115g) frozen chopped onions

2 cups (350g) frozen sliced peppers

4 spring onions, sliced

250g frozen raw king prawns (defrosted on the day you want to serve the stir-fry)

For the sauce:

4 tbsp low-sodium soy sauce

1 tbsp sweet chilli sauce (shop-bought or see page 215)

1 tbsp sesame oil

1 tbsp cornflour

1 tsp frozen chopped ginger

1 tsp frozen chopped garlic

To serve

Lighter Serve: Scattered with sesame seeds and fresh coriander

Family Serve: On a bed of egg noodles, scattered with sesame seeds and fresh coriander

1 To make the sauce, put all the ingredients in a small bowl and whisk to combine. Set aside.

TO COOK

Heat the oil in a wok or large frying pan over a medium-high heat. Add all the vegetables and stir-fry for 4–5 minutes, until starting to soften. Add the sauce and defrosted prawns to the pan and continue to stir-fry for around 5 minutes, until the prawns are cooked through and the sauce has thickened. If the sauce is too thick, add a splash of water to loosen. Serve hot.

TO FREEZE

Working quickly to ensure that the frozen ingredients do not start to defrost, add the prawns and all of the vegetables to a large, labelled freezer bag. Transfer the stir-fry sauce to a smaller, labelled freezer bag and freeze flat, both alongside each other, in the freezer for up to 3 months.

TO COOK FROM FROZEN

Remove the frozen stir-fry mix and sauce from the freezer and leave to defrost in the fridge, ideally overnight. Once defrosted, pour off any excess water from the bag with the prawns and vegetables, then cook the stir-fry as described in the *To Cook* section, left.

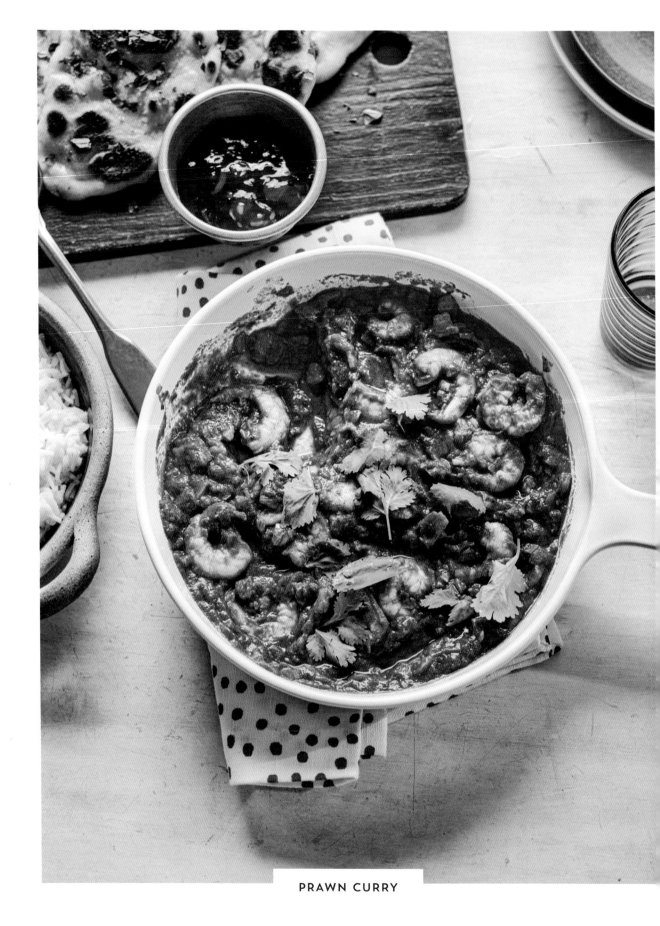

PRAWN CURRY

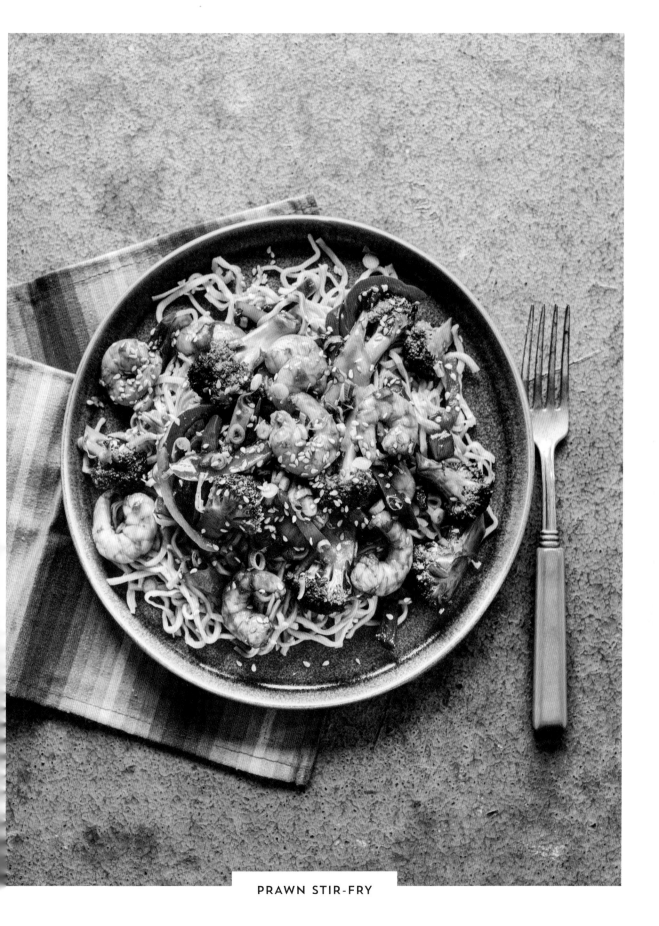

PRAWN STIR-FRY

CHICKPEA & SWEET POTATO CURRY

PREP: 5 MINS **COOK:** 40 MINS **SERVES:** 4 **SUGAR:** 17G **KCAL:** 484

This wholesome curry is mild and fragrant, rather than hot and spicy, and is further lifted by the addition of sweet potato, meaning that the whole family will love it. If you like more heat, feel free to ramp up the spice to suit your tastes, but I find that this is the perfect balance that keeps everyone, from the spice-averse to the chilli-heads, more than happy.

low-calorie cooking spray
1 cup (115g) frozen chopped onions
1 tsp frozen chopped garlic
2 cups (300g) frozen sweet
  potato chunks
1 tbsp curry powder
1 tsp ground cumin
2 x 400g cans chopped tomatoes
2 x 400g cans chickpeas, drained
1 tbsp tomato purée
1 x 400g can reduced-fat
  coconut milk
salt and freshly ground pepper

To serve

Lighter Serve: Cauliflower rice (p.203).
Family Serve: Basmati rice, Light-And-Easy Naan Breads (p.208) and mango chutney

1 Spray a large saucepan with low-calorie cooking spray and place over a medium heat. Add the onions and garlic and cook, stirring continuously, for 2–3 minutes until soft.

2 Add the sweet potato chunks, curry powder and cumin and stir to combine, then add the chopped tomatoes, drained chickpeas, tomato purée and coconut milk and stir again. Bring to the boil, then reduce the heat to a gentle simmer and leave to cook for around 35 minutes, until the sweet potatoes are tender and the sauce has reduced and thickened slightly.

If you are also making the Turkey Keema Matar, prepare this while the curry is cooking.

TO SERVE

Once the curry is cooked, season to taste with salt and pepper, then serve with your choice of accompaniments alongside.

TO FREEZE

Once cooked, season the curry to taste, then set aside to cool to room temperature. Once cooled, ladle the curry into a large, labelled, freezer bag and freeze flat for up to 3 months.

TO REHEAT FROM FROZEN

Remove the bag from the freezer and leave to completely defrost in the fridge, ideally overnight. Once defrosted, pour the contents into a large saucepan and place over a medium heat for 10–15 minutes, stirring occasionally, until piping hot all of the way through. Serve.

TURKEY KEEMA MATAR

PREP: 10 MINS **COOK:** 25 MINS **SERVES:** 4 **SUGAR:** 9.4G **KCAL:** 303

Keema Matar is a delicious, delicately spiced Indian curry made with minced meat and peas. Using lean turkey mince as opposed to beef or lamb is a great way to bring down the fat and calorie content of the dish without compromising on any of the taste.

low-calorie cooking spray
1 cup (115g) frozen chopped onions
1 tsp frozen chopped garlic
2 tsp frozen chopped ginger
500g lean turkey mince
1 tbsp mild curry powder
2 tsp ground cumin
2 tbsp tomato purée
1½ cups (360ml) low-sodium chicken stock
2 cups (310g) frozen peas

To serve
Lighter Serve: Cauliflower Rice (p.203)
Family Serve: Basmati rice, Light-And-Easy Naan Breads (p.208) and mango chutney

1 Spray a large saucepan with low-calorie cooking spray and place over a medium heat. Add the onions, garlic and ginger and cook, stirring continuously, for 2–3 minutes until soft.
2 Add the turkey mince, breaking it up with a wooden spoon, and cook, stirring regularly, until browned.
3 Add the curry powder, cumin, tomato purée and chicken stock and cook, stirring occasionally, for 10 minutes.

> If you are cooking both dishes, use this time to wipe down your counters and prepare any freezer bags for storing your meals.

4 After 10 minutes, add the frozen peas to the pan and stir to combine. Cook for 5 minutes more, until the peas are tender.

TO SERVE

The curry is now ready to serve with your choice of accompaniments.

TO FREEZE

Remove the pan from the heat and set aside until the curry has cooled to room temperature. Transfer the cooled curry to a large, labelled freezer bag and freeze flat for up to 3 months.

TO REHEAT FROM FROZEN

This can be defrosted in the fridge overnight and then reheated in a pan until piping hot, or reheated from frozen. If reheating from frozen, tip the frozen Keema Matar mixture into a large saucepan, cover with a lid and place over a low heat. Cook the mixture, removing the lid occasionally and breaking it up with a wooden spoon as the mixture defrosts, until it is fully defrosted and piping hot all of the way through. Serve hot with your choice of accompaniments.

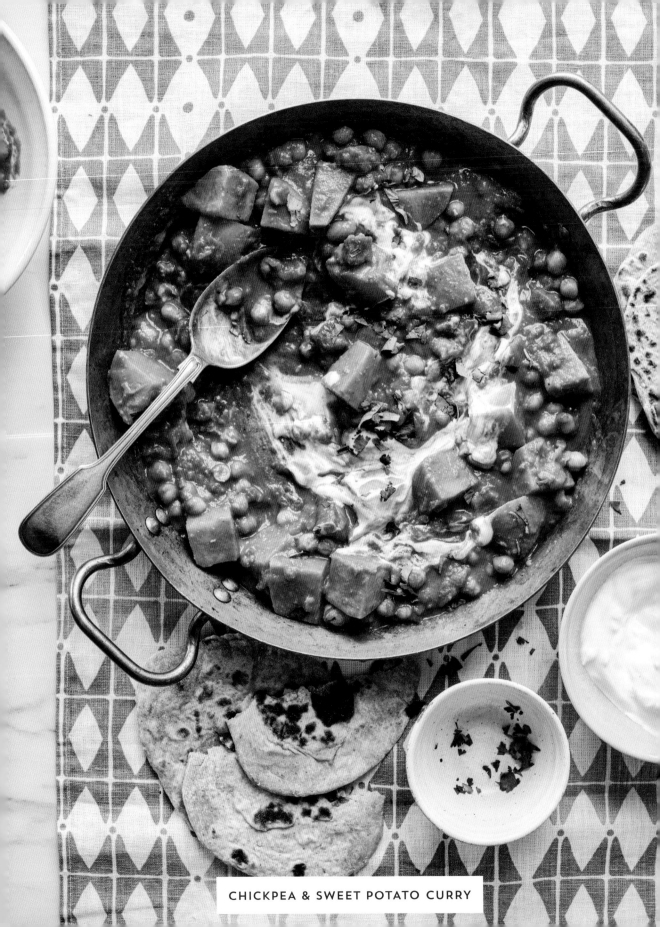

CHICKPEA & SWEET POTATO CURRY

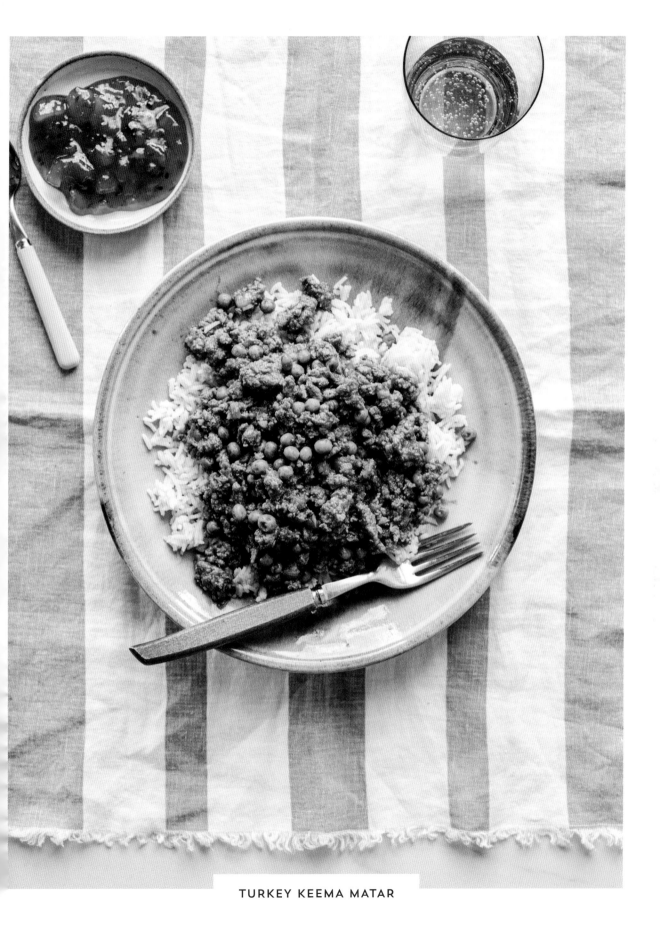

TURKEY KEEMA MATAR

CHINESE 5-SPICE PORK LOIN

PREP: 5 MINS **COOK:** 20–25 MINS **SERVES:** 4 **SUGAR:** 4.4G **KCAL:** 230

The sauce for this Chinese-inspired pork dish is packed with flavour and contains just three ingredients, all of which can be found in a well-stocked storecupboard. The pork loin is cooked whole, then sliced, so making it in advance for the freezer requires minimal preparation. Quicker, simpler, healthier and far kinder on the wallet than reaching for that Chinese-takeaway menu!

1 tsp Chinese five spice
3 tbsp hoisin sauce
1 tsp garlic granules
1 large pork tenderloin fillet
   (500–550g), white fat trimmed
low-calorie cooking spray

To serve
Lighter Serve: Cauliflower Rice
(p.203), pak choi and mange tout
Family Serve: Brown Basmati
Rice, pak choi and mange tout

1   Add the Chinese five spice, hoisin sauce and garlic granules to a small bowl and stir to combine.

TO COOK

Lay the pork tenderloin on a foil-lined baking tray and pour over the sauce, using your hands to make sure the meat is well coated in the sauce. Spray lightly with low-calorie cooking spray, then transfer to an oven preheated to 180°C/350°F/gas mark 4 and cook for 20–25 minutes, until sticky, golden and cooked all of the way through. Rest for 5 minutes, then slice and serve.

TO FREEZE

Put the uncooked pork tenderloin in a large, labelled freezer bag and pour over the sauce. Massage the sides of the bag to ensure the meat is well coated in the sauce, then seal and freeze flat for up to 3 months.

TO COOK FROM FROZEN

Remove the bag of marinated pork from the freezer and leave to defrost fully in the fridge, ideally overnight. Once defrosted, transfer the pork to a foil-lined baking tray and cook as described in the *To Cook* section, left.

CHINESE 5-SPICE CHICKEN

PREP: 10 MINS **COOK:** 20-30 MINS **SERVES:** 4 **SUGAR:** 13G **KCAL:** 278

This Chinese-inspired chicken dish is a twist on the delicious *char siu* pork that is found in many restaurants. The quick marinade is packed with flavour and easily knocked up from storecupboard staples, which helps keep the shopping list nice and short!

2 tsp frozen chopped garlic
2 tsp frozen chopped ginger
2 tsp Chinese 5 spice
4 tbsp low-sodium soy sauce
1 tbsp white wine vinegar
2 tbsp runny honey
1 tbsp reduced-salt-and-sugar
   tomato ketchup
6-8 skinless, boneless chicken
   thighs

To serve

Lighter Serve: Cauliflower rice
(p.203) and mange tout
Harissa Sauce (p.137)
spooned over
Family Serve: Wholewheat
noodles and mange tout

1 Combine the garlic, ginger, Chinese 5 spice, soy sauce, white wine vinegar, honey and ketchup in a large bowl.

TO COOK

If you are making this to serve now, add the chicken thighs to the bowl and stir to combine with the marinade. Set aside to marinate for 20 minutes. Preheat the oven to 180°C/350°F/gas mark 4. Once marinated, pour the chicken into a roasting tin and transfer to the oven to cook for 20–25 minutes, until cooked through, sticky and delicious. Serve hot.

TO FREEZE

Place the raw chicken in a large, labelled, reusable freezer bag and pour over the marinade. Massage the bag with your hands to make sure the chicken is well coated, then seal the bag, expelling any air, and freeze flat for up to 3 months.

TO COOK FROM FROZEN

Remove the bag from the freezer and leave to completely defrost in the fridge, ideally overnight. Once defrosted, pour the contents into a roasting tin and spread out in an even layer. Transfer to an oven preheated to 180°C/350°F/gas mark 4 and cook as described in the *To Cook* section, left.

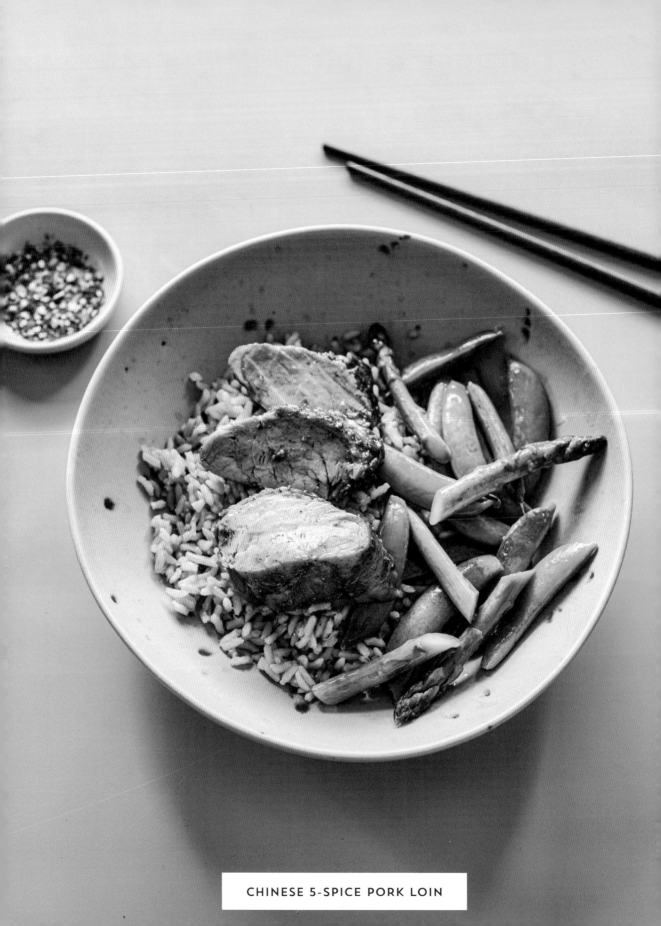

CHINESE 5-SPICE PORK LOIN

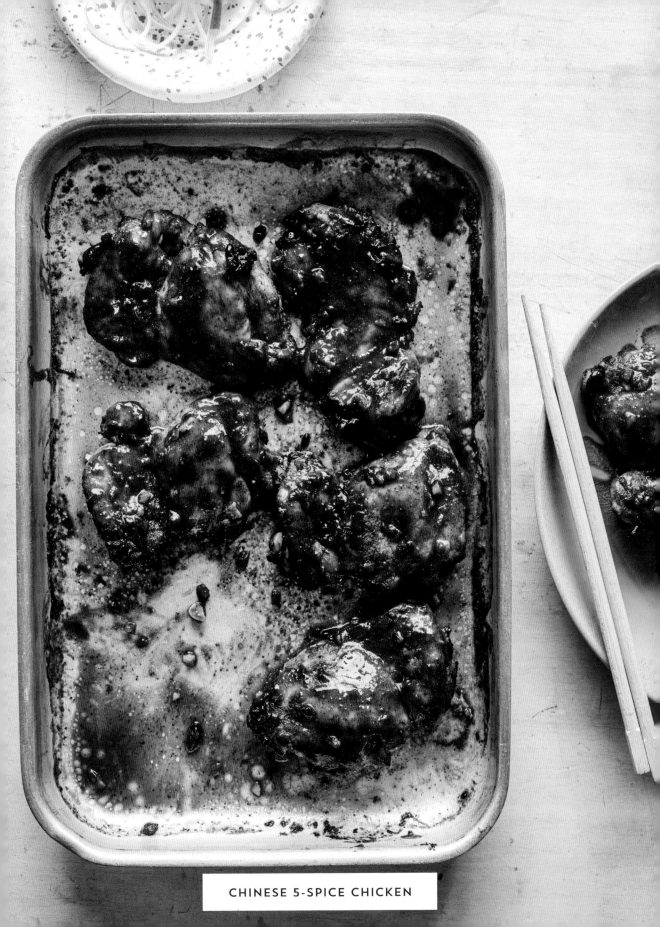

CHINESE 5-SPICE CHICKEN

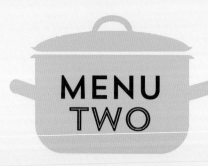

MENU TWO

3 FOR THE FRIDGE,

3 FOR THE FREEZER

Are you ready to batch three family meals for the week ahead and three to store in the freezer for another time in just 45 minutes? You will be making three recipes, each of which is doubled-up to feed eight people, so you simply need to split the recipe into two family meals before freezing one and putting the other in the fridge for the week ahead. The recipes are a mixture of cooked and no-cook freezer-bag meals, so while one recipe is bubbling away on the stove or cooking in the oven, you can be making the next meal ready for the fridge and freezer.

The shopping list on the opposite page includes everything you need and I have scaled up the ingredients for you so you don't need to worry about doubling the recipe. Simply buy what's on the shopping list and you will have everything you need to make the six meals. Once you have your shopping, lay the ingredients out into piles according to the groupings overleaf, so you have exactly what you need for each recipe to hand. Then simply follow the numbered guide and you can't go wrong!

Don't panic if this takes you more than 45 minutes the first time you cook it – you will get quicker each time you make it. So, roll up your sleeves, get cooking and think about the time you will be saving yourself in the future!

YOU WILL BE MAKING:

SWEET & SOUR CHICKEN
KUNG PAO PORK
THAI SEA BASS PARCELS

SHOPPING LIST

Fresh

4 skinless, boneless chicken breasts

4 large carrots

2 bunches spring onions

2 onions

4 red peppers

1kg lean, diced pork

500g pack pak choi

8 sea bass fillets

Frozen

1 x 75g bag frozen chopped garlic

1 x 75g bag frozen chopped ginger

1 x 500g bag frozen chopped onions

1 x 500g bag frozen sliced peppers

Storecupboard

1 x 500g pack cornflour

1 x 250ml bottle low-sodium soy sauce

1 x 340g bottle runny honey

1 x 350ml bottle white wine vinegar

1 x 400g can pineapple chunks in juice

low-calorie cooking spray

1 x 350g bottle sweet chilli sauce

2 low-sodium chicken stock cubes

1 small pot lemongrass paste

INGREDIENTS

GET ORGANISED! Before you start cooking, make sure that your kitchen surfaces are cleared down, then lay all the ingredients out in individual piles according to the groupings below.

SWEET & SOUR CHICKEN

4 skinless, boneless chicken breasts, cut into bite-sized pieces
4 tbsp cornflour
4 tbsp low-sodium soy sauce
4 tbsp runny honey
4 tbsp white wine vinegar
4 tsp frozen chopped garlic
2 tsp frozen chopped ginger
1 x 400g can pineapple chunks, drained and juice reserved
low-calorie cooking spray
2 cups (230g) frozen chopped onions
2 large carrots, peeled and cut into matchsticks
4 cups (700g) frozen sliced peppers

KUNG PAO PORK

8 tbsp low-sodium soy sauce
4 tbsp cornflour
2 tbsp white wine vinegar
4 tbsp sweet chilli sauce
8 spring onions, finely sliced
2 tsp frozen chopped garlic
low-calorie cooking spray
2 onions, finely sliced
4 red peppers, deseeded and finely sliced
2 large carrots, peeled and cut into matchsticks
1kg lean, diced pork
2 cups (480ml) low-sodium chicken stock

THAI SEA BASS PARCELS

4 tsp frozen chopped garlic
4 tsp frozen chopped ginger
2 tsp lemongrass paste
3–4 tbsp sweet chilli sauce
8 spring onions, finely sliced
10 tbsp low-sodium soy sauce
500g pak choi
8 sea bass fillets
you will also need 8 30x25cm (12x10in) rectangles of foil

METHOD

SWEET & SOUR CHICKEN

1 Put the chopped chicken breasts into a mixing bowl and sprinkle over 2 tablespoons of the cornflour, turning the chicken in the cornflour to ensure it is well coated.

2 In a separate bowl, combine the remaining 2 tablespoons of cornflour with the soy sauce, honey, white wine vinegar, garlic, ginger and the reserved juice from the can of pineapple chunks. Stir to combine and set aside.

3 Spray a frying pan with low-calorie cooking spray and place over a medium heat. Add the onions, carrots and cornflour-coated chicken and cook, stirring continuously, for 5 minutes.

4 Add the peppers and pineapple chunks to the pan and continue to cook, stirring, for 3 minutes, until the peppers have softened.

5 Pour over the sauce and leave to cook, stirring occasionally, for 5 minutes, until the sauce is thick and glossy. Remove from the heat and set aside to cool.

KUNG PAO PORK

6 Put the soy sauce, cornflour, white wine vinegar, sweet chilli sauce, spring onions and garlic in a small bowl and stir to combine. Set aside.

7 Spray a frying pan with low-calorie cooking spray and place over a medium heat. Add the onions, sliced peppers, carrots and diced pork and leave to cook, stirring occasionally, for around 8 minutes, until the pork is cooked through and the vegetables have softened.

THAI SEA BASS PARCELS

8 Put the garlic, ginger, lemongrass paste, sweet chilli sauce, spring onions and soy sauce in a small bowl and stir to combine. Set aside.

9 Lay your 8 rectangles of foil next to each other on the kitchen counter. Pull the leaves from the pak choi and distribute equally between the foil rectangles, placing the leaves in the centre of each rectangle.

10 Lay a seabass fillet on top of each pile of leaves.

11 Spoon the sauce over the sea bass fillets, dividing it equally between each fillet. Bring up the sides of each sheet of foil and scrunch together to form a well-sealed parcel.

12 Place 4 parcels each in 2 large, labelled freezer bags. Transfer 1 of the bags to the freezer for up to 3 months. Transfer the other bag to the fridge to use in the coming week. Make sure you label the bag for the fridge with the use-by date of the sea bass, so that you know when it has to be used by.

CONTINUED OVERLEAF...

SWEET & SOUR CHICKEN CONTINUED...

13 Once the Sweet & Sour Chicken has cooled to room temperature, divide it between 2 large, labelled freezer bags and add half of the sauce to each bag. Freeze one flat in the freezer for up to 3 months and keep the other in the fridge to use in the week ahead.

KUNG PAO PORK CONTINED...

14 Once the Kung Pao Pork has cooled to room temperature, divide it between 2 large, labelled freezer bags. Freeze one flat in the freezer for up to 3 months and keep the other in the fridge to use in the week ahead.

Congratulations!
You have just made six meals!
Three for the week ahead
and three for the freezer.

WHEN YOU COME TO COOK

Once cooked, all of these meals are best fully defrosted before cooking. All reheated meals should reach a temperature of 74°C/165°F. Always make sure any reheated food is piping hot before serving. Cooking instructions for each dish are given below.

SWEET & SOUR CHICKEN

FROM THE FRIDGE

Reheat the chicken in a saucepan over a medium heat until piping hot, or transfer to a microwaveable bowl and heat on high for 5–6 minutes, until piping hot. If the sauce is too thick, add a splash of water to loosen.

FROM THE FREEZER

Remove the chicken from the freezer and leave to fully defrost in the fridge, ideally overnight. Once defrosted, reheat the chicken in a saucepan over a medium heat until piping hot, or transfer to a microwavable bowl and heat on high for 5–6 minutes, until piping hot. If the sauce is too thick, add a splash of water to loosen.

To serve
Lighter Serve: Cauliflower Rice (p.203)
Family Serve: Basmati rice and prawn crackers

KUNG PAO PORK

FROM THE FRIDGE

Reheat the pork in a saucepan over a medium heat until piping hot, or transfer to a microwavable bowl and heat on high for 5–6 minutes, until piping hot. If the sauce is too thick, add a splash of water to loosen.

FROM THE FREEZER

Remove the pork from the freezer and leave to fully defrost in the fridge, ideally overnight. Once defrosted, reheat the pork in a saucepan over a medium heat until piping hot, or transfer to a microwavable bowl and heat on high for 5–6 minutes, until piping hot. If the sauce is too thick, add a splash of water to loosen.

To serve
Lighter Serve: Cauliflower Rice (p.203) and a sprinkling of unsalted cashew nuts
Family Serve: Basmati rice and a sprinkling of unsalted cashew nuts

THAI SEA BASS PARCELS

FROM THE FRIDGE

Preheat the oven to 180°C/350°F/gas mark 4. Lay the parcels on a baking tray and transfer to the oven for 15 minutes, until the sea bass is cooked through. Open the parcels and transfer the contents to serving plates. Serve hot.

FROM THE FREEZER

Remove the sea bass parcels from the freezer and leave to fully defrost in the fridge, ideally overnight. Once defrosted, preheat the oven to 180°C/350°F/gas mark 4. Lay the parcels on a baking tray and transfer to the oven for 15 minutes, until the sea bass is cooked through. Open the parcels and transfer the contents to serving plates. Serve hot.

To serve
Lighter Serve: Steamed green vegetables
Family Serve: Wholewheat noodles and steamed green vegetables

WEEKNIGHTS

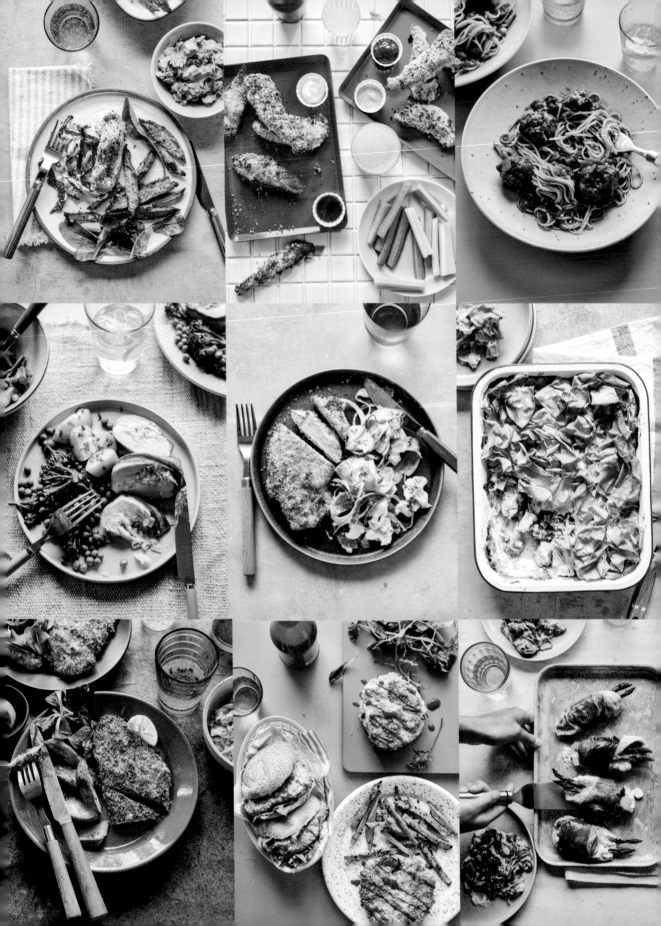

WEEKNIGHTS

Monday—Friday cooking is the backbone of any home cook's repertoire.
The recipes in this chapter are all simple and speedy, but are sure to keep
the whole family happy after long days at school or work. As ever, they
can all be made ahead and stored in the freezer until they are needed, and
many can be cooked straight from frozen. But, even if you want to make
these fresh, they can be on the table with minimum fuss.

One-pan meals are great for midweek cooking, as you can just put
everything in a tin, put it in the oven and get on with something else and
half an hour later you've got a tasty dinner ready to go. My Chicken,
Butter Bean & Leek Bake (p.122) and Harissa Cauliflower Traybake
(p.137) are both great examples of this low-fuss, flavour-packed type of
cooking. For a midweek showstopper, my Chicken & Chorizo Filo Pie
(p.118) is topped with light and easy filo pastry and is far easier to put
together than it looks. You will also find lighter versions of hearty family
classics, such as shepherd's pie, chilli and meatballs.

The trend for hearty family favourites continues in the *3 for the Fridge,
3 for the Freezer* section (p.150—155) , where you will find delicious, no-
fuss recipes for a Turkey Bolognese, Thai Chicken Noodle Soup and a
Lamb Meatloaf.

CHICKEN & CHORIZO FILO PIE

PREP: 25 MINS **COOK:** 25–30 MINS **SERVES:** 6 **SUGAR:** 8.6G **KCAL:** 434

Filo pastry makes a great alternative to more traditional shortcrust in this chicken pie, as it is both lighter and lower calorie as well as melding well with the subtle spice of the chorizo used in the filling. If making this ahead to store in the freezer, freeze the filo pastry next to the filling so that you can easily defrost both at the same.

low calorie cooking spray

1 cup (115g) frozen chopped onions

1 tsp frozen chopped garlic

3 skinless, boneless chicken breasts, cut into bite-sized pieces

⅔ cup (75g) ready-diced chorizo

1 tsp smoked paprika

1 red pepper, diced

1 orange pepper, diced

2 tbsp plain flour

1½ cups (360ml) low-sodium chicken stock

2 tbsp reduced-fat crème fraîche

½ cup (30g) low-fat, pre-grated cheddar cheese

10 sheets filo pastry

To serve

Lighter Serve: Steamed green veg
Family Serve: Piri-Piri Sweet Potato Chips (p.205) and steamed green veg

1 Spray a large frying pan with low-calorie cooking spray and place over a medium heat. Add the onions, garlic, diced chicken, chorizo, paprika and diced peppers and cook, stirring frequently, for around 10 minutes until the chicken is cooked through and the onions are soft and translucent.

2 Add the flour to the pan and stir to coat the chicken and onion mixture, then gradually pour in the chicken stock, stirring and thickening the sauce between each addition, until all of the stock is used up. Bring the mixture to the boil, then reduce the heat to a simmer and leave to cook, stirring occasionally, for 10 minutes.

> If you are also making the Cheesy Cajun-Pepper-Stuffed Chicken, assemble this while the pie filling is cooking.

3 Remove the pan from the heat and stir through the crème fraîche and grated cheese.

TO COOK

Transfer the pie filling to a large baking dish, then scrunch the filo sheets into rosettes and place over the filling. Spray the pastry with low-calorie cooking spray, then transfer the pie to an oven preheated to 180°C/350°F/gas mark 4 for 25–30 minutes, until the pastry is crisp and golden.

TO FREEZE

Set the pie filling aside to cool to room temperature, then transfer to a labelled freezer bag and freeze flat for up to 3 months. For ease of assembly after defrosting, I like to freeze the filling alongside the filo so that both can be removed from the freezer at the same time.

TO COOK FROM FROZEN

Remove the pie filling and pastry from the freezer and leave to fully defrost, ideally overnight in the fridge. Transfer the pie filling to a large baking dish and top with the pastry and cook as described in the *To Cook* section, left.

CHEESY CAJUN-PEPPER-STUFFED CHICKEN

PREP: 5 MINS **COOK:** 25 MINS **SERVES:** 4 **SUGAR:** 3.5G **KCAL:** 223

Punchy Cajun spices combine with a rich and tangy cheese sauce in this stuffed chicken breast that is packed with flavour but surprisingly low in fat. If you are making these for the freezer, be sure to work fast and get them back in the freezer as quickly as possible so that the frozen peppers don't defrost as you are assembling the dish.

4 tbsp low-fat cream cheese
½ cup (30g) low-fat, pre-grated cheddar cheese
3 tsp Cajun seasoning
4 skinless, boneless chicken breasts
4 handfuls frozen sliced peppers
low-calorie cooking spray
salt and freshly ground pepper

To serve
Lighter Serve: Leafy green salad
Family Serve: Piri-Piri Sweet Potato Chips (p.205) and a leafy green salad

1 Put the cream cheese, grated cheddar and 2 teaspoons of the Cajun seasoning in a small bowl and stir to combine. Set aside.
2 Place a chicken breast flat on a chopping board and press down with the palm of your hand. Working from the thickest end of the breast, insert a sharp knife two-thirds of the way through the meat and carefully slice down the length to the thinnest end to create a pocket.
3 Repeat with the remaining chicken breasts.
4 Spoon a quarter of the spiced cheese mixture into the pocket of each chicken breast and top with a handful of frozen sliced peppers. Close the chicken breasts over the filling and season with salt, pepper and the remaining teaspoon of Cajun seasoning. Spray each chicken breast with a couple of sprays of low-calorie cooking spray.

TO COOK

Transfer to a foil-lined baking tray and cook in an oven preheated to 180°C/350°F/gas mark 4 for 25–30 minutes, until cooked through, tender and juicy.

TO FREEZE

Transfer the uncooked stuffed chicken breasts to a labelled freezer bag and freeze flat for up to 3 months.

TO COOK FROM FROZEN

Remove the stuffed chicken breasts from the freezer and leave to defrost fully in the fridge, ideally overnight, then cook as described in the *To Cook* section, left.

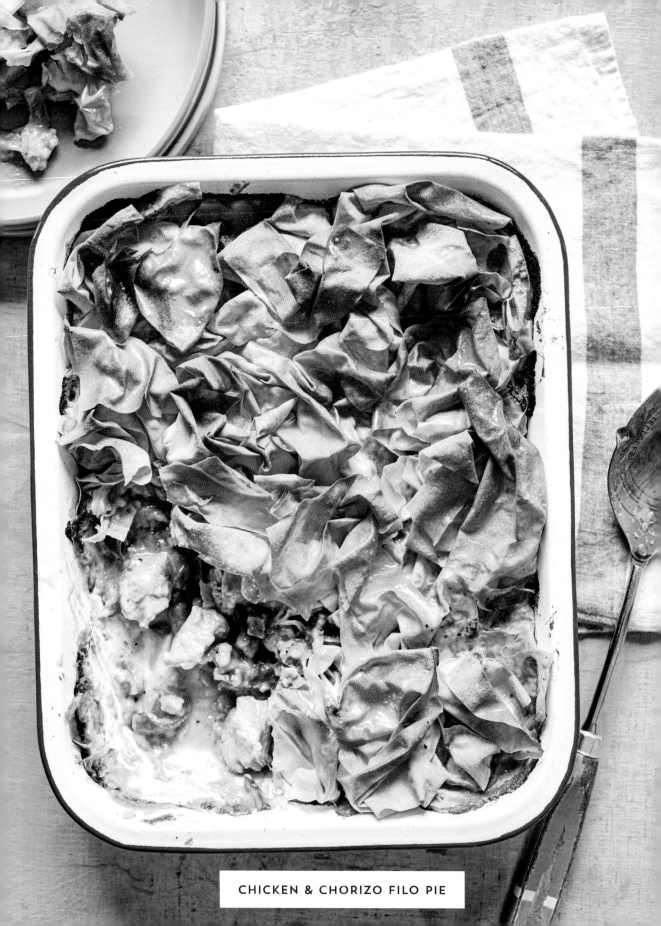

CHICKEN & CHORIZO FILO PIE

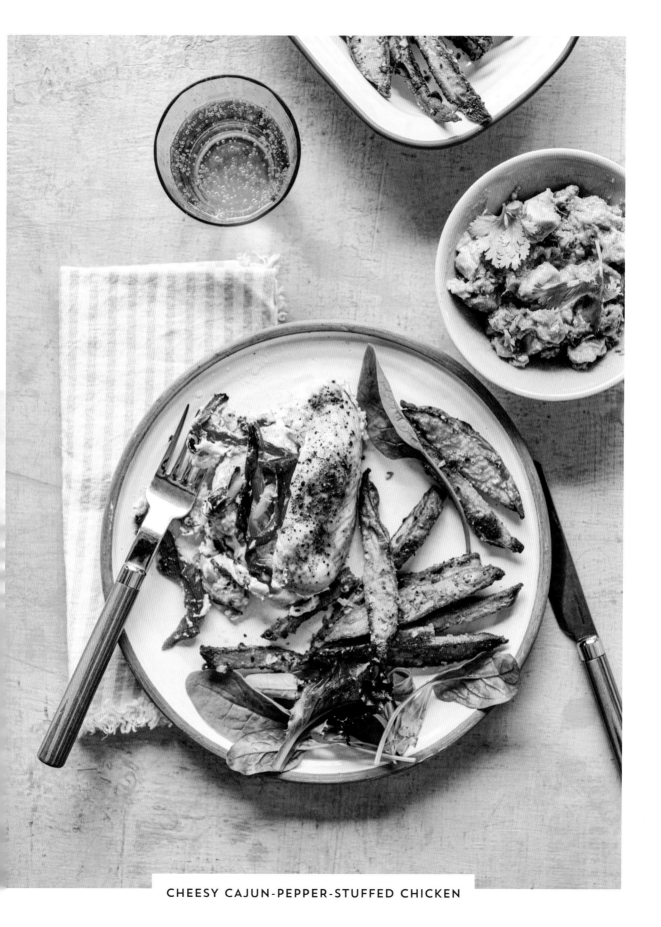

CHEESY CAJUN-PEPPER-STUFFED CHICKEN

CHICKEN, BUTTER BEAN & LEEK BAKE

PREP: 10 MINS **COOK:** 40-45 MINS **SERVES:** 4 **SUGAR:** 3.6G **KCAL:** 222

4–6 skinless, boneless chicken
  thighs
1 x 400g can butter beans,
  drained
3 medium leeks, chopped
2 tsp frozen chopped garlic
1 handful fresh tarragon leaves,
  finely chopped (or 1 tsp dried
  tarragon)
juice of 1 lemon
2 tbsp olive oil, plus extra for
  drizzling
salt and freshly ground pepper
8–10 cherry tomatoes, to serve

To serve

Lighter Serve: New potatoes and
steamed green vegetables
Family Serve: Buttered new
potatoes and veg of your choice

TO COOK

Preheat the oven to 180°C/350°F/
gas mark 4. Lay the chicken thighs
in the base of a large baking dish
in an even layer, then scatter over
the butter beans and leeks. Add
the garlic and herbs to the pan,
then pour over the lemon juice and
season with salt and pepper. Drizzle
over the 2 tablespoons of olive
oil, then mix everything with your
hands to combine. Transfer to the
oven for 40–45 minutes, until the
chicken is golden, juicy and cooked
through. Scatter over the cherry
tomatoes to serve.

TO FREEZE

Place all of the raw ingredients,
except the cherry tomatoes, in a
large, labelled, reusable freezer bag
and massage gently with your hands
to make sure everything is well
combined. Seal the bag, expelling
any air, and freeze flat for up to
3 months.

TO COOK FROM FROZEN

Remove the bag from the freezer
and leave to completely defrost in
the fridge, ideally overnight. Once
defrosted, put the contents into a
roasting tin and drizzle with a little
extra olive oil. Transfer to an oven
preheated to 180°C/350°F/gas
mark 4 and cook as described in the
To Cook section, left.

PORK SCHNITZEL

PREP: 10 MINS **COOK:** 15–20 MINS **SERVES:** 4 **SUGAR:** 1.2G **KCAL:** 538

With its crunchy, golden crust yielding to wonderfully tender meat, schnitzel is such a treat.
I like to have a stash of these in the freezer as they can be cooked directly from frozen for a
speedy-but-tasty midweek meal with minimal effort on my part.

1 cup (110g) plain flour
2 cups (90g) panko breadcrumbs
1 tsp garlic salt
½ cup (50g) pre-grated Parmesan
  cheese
2 eggs, beaten
4 boneless pork loin steaks, fat
  trimmed
low-calorie cooking spray
salt and freshly ground pepper

To serve
Lighter Serve: Low-fat coleslaw
and salad
Family Serve: Coleslaw, potato
wedges and corn on the cob

1   Put the flour in a wide, shallow bowl. Put the panko breadcrumbs, garlic
    salt and Parmesan in a second bowl and season with a generous grinding
    of salt and pepper. Put the beaten eggs into a third bowl, then set all
    3 dishes next to each other on the worktop.
2   Lay the pork steaks flat on a chopping board, cover with clingfilm, then
    press down with a large, flat-bottomed object, such as a saucepan, to
    flatten slightly. You are aiming for a thickness of around 3cm (1¼in).
3   Working with one pork steak at a time, dredge the pork in the flour,
    shaking off any excess, then dip in the egg and, finally, press into the
    spiced panko breadcrumbs until coated. Set aside and repeat until all
    4 pork loin steaks are coated.

TO COOK

Lay the coated pork steaks on a
lined baking tray and spray each
one 4–5 times with low-calorie
cooking spray. Transfer to an
oven preheated to 180°C/350°F/
gas mark 4 and cook for 15–20
minutes, until golden brown and
cooked all of the way through.

TO FREEZE

Transfer the uncooked schnitzel
to a large, labelled freezer bag and
freeze flat for up to 3 months.

TO COOK FROM FROZEN

These can be cooked directly from
frozen. Lay the frozen schnitzel on
a lined baking tray and spray each
one 4–5 times with low-calorie
cooking spray. Transfer to an
oven preheated to 180°C/350°F/
gas mark 4 and cook for 25–30
minutes, until golden brown and
piping hot all of the way through.

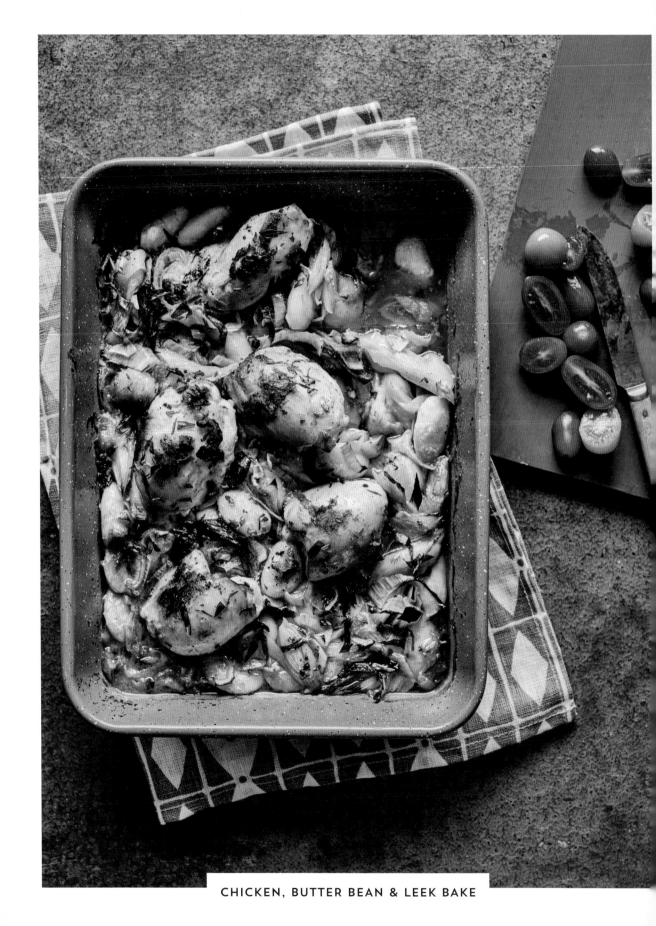

CHICKEN, BUTTER BEAN & LEEK BAKE

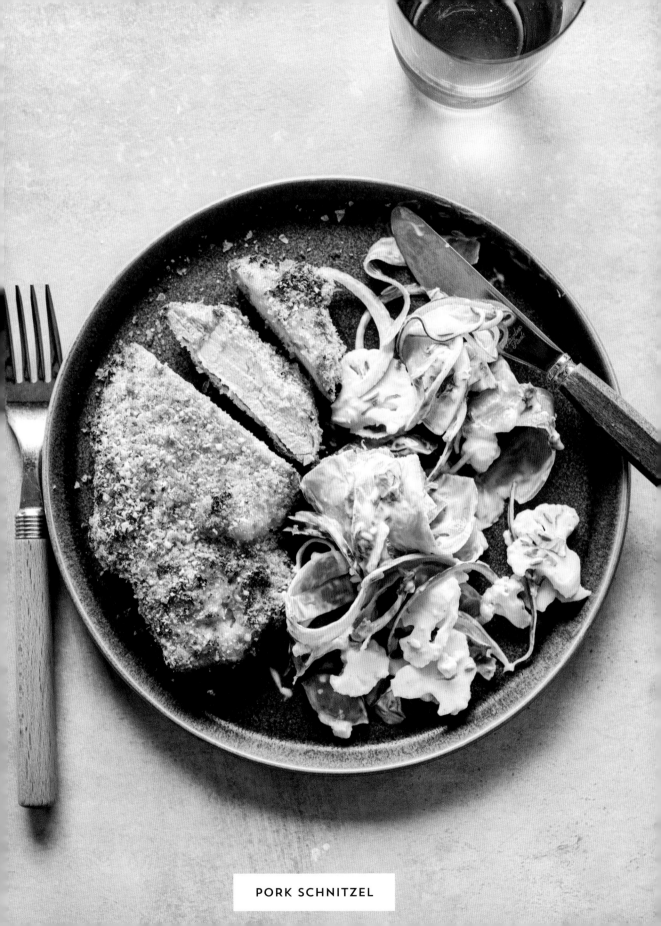

PORK SCHNITZEL

LOW-FAT CHICKEN GOUJONS

PREP: 10 MINS **COOK:** 25-30 MINS **SERVES:** 4 **SUGAR:** 1.1G **KCAL:** 388

These wonderfully crispy goujons are baked rather than fried, which reduces the calories but keeps the same great taste! Kids will love these, but they can be dressed up with your favourite sauces to make them a hit with the adults in your family, too. The method for making these is almost identical to the Fajita-Spiced Chicken Schnitzel recipe (opposite) so I like to make both at the same time.

1 cup (110g) plain flour
2 cups (90g) panko breadcrumbs
3 eggs
4 skinless, boneless chicken
  breasts, cut into long strips
low-calorie cooking spray
salt and freshly ground pepper

To serve

Lighter Serve: Green leafy salad and your choice of dressing (p.210–11)
Family Serve: Skin-On Chips (p.204) and peas

1 Put the flour in a shallow bowl. Put the panko breadcrumbs in a second bowl and season with a generous grinding of salt and pepper. Crack the eggs into a third bowl and beat with a fork, then set all 3 bowls next to each other on the worktop.
2 Working with one strip of chicken at a time, dredge the chicken in the flour, shaking off any excess, then dip in the egg and, finally, roll in the panko breadcrumbs until coated. Set aside on a baking parchment-lined baking tray and repeat until all of the chicken strips are coated.

TO COOK

Spray each goujon 2–3 times with low-calorie cooking spray. Transfer the baking tray to an oven preheated to 180°C/350°F/gas mark 4 and cook for 25–30 minutes, until golden brown and cooked all of the way through.

TO FREEZE

Transfer the uncooked goujons on the baking tray to the freezer for 1 hour to allow them to firm up, then transfer to a large, labelled freezer bag and freeze flat for up to 3 months.

TO COOK FROM FROZEN

These can be cooked directly from frozen. Lay the frozen goujons on a baking parchment-lined baking tray and spray each one 2–3 times with low-calorie cooking spray. Transfer to an oven preheated to 180°C/350°F/gas mark 4 and cook for 30 minutes, until golden brown and piping hot all of the way through.

FAJITA-SPICED CHICKEN SCHNITZEL

PREP: 10-15 MINS **COOK:** 30 MINS **SERVES:** 4 **SUGAR:** 2.1G **KCAL:** 381

These deceptively healthy Fajita-Spiced Chicken Schnitzels feel like a treat and are sure to be a hit with the whole family. If you're an experienced batcher, it's worth doubling or tripling the recipe and making a big batch of these, as they can be served in lots of different ways to feel fresh and new time after time.

1 cup (110g) plain flour
2 cups (90g) panko breadcrumbs
1 tsp garlic powder
2 tsp fajita seasoning
3 eggs, beaten
4 skinless, boneless chicken
   breasts
low-calorie cooking spray
salt and freshly ground pepper

To serve
Lighter Serve: Low-fat coleslaw and salad
Family Serve: Skin-On Chips (p.204), coleslaw and salad

> If you have already made the Low-Fat Chicken Goujons, use the same bowls to bread your chicken, adding the additional flavourings to the panko bowl for this dish.

1 Put the flour in a shallow bowl. Put the panko breadcrumbs, garlic powder and fajita seasoning in a second bowl and season with a generous grinding of salt and pepper. Put the beaten eggs into a third bowl, then set all 3 dishes next to each other on the worktop.
2 Lay the chicken breasts flat on a chopping board, cover with clingfilm, then press down with a large, flat-bottomed object, such as a saucepan, to flatten slightly. You are aiming for a thickness of around 3cm (1¼in).
3 Working with one chicken breast at a time, dredge the chicken in the flour, shaking off any excess, then dip in the egg and, finally, press into the spiced panko breadcrumbs until coated. Set aside and repeat until all 4 breasts are coated.

TO COOK

Lay the coated chicken breasts on a lined baking tray and spray each one 4–5 times with low-calorie cooking spray. Transfer to an oven preheated to 180°C/350°F/gas mark 4 and cook for 25–30 minutes, until golden brown and cooked all of the way through.

TO FREEZE

Transfer the uncooked coated chicken breasts to a large, labelled freezer bag and freeze flat for up to 3 months.

TO COOK FROM FROZEN

These can be cooked directly from frozen. Lay the frozen, coated chicken breasts on a lined baking tray and spray each one 4–5 times with low-calorie cooking spray. Transfer to an oven preheated to 180°C/350°F/gas mark 4 and cook for 35–40 minutes, until golden brown and piping hot all of the way through.

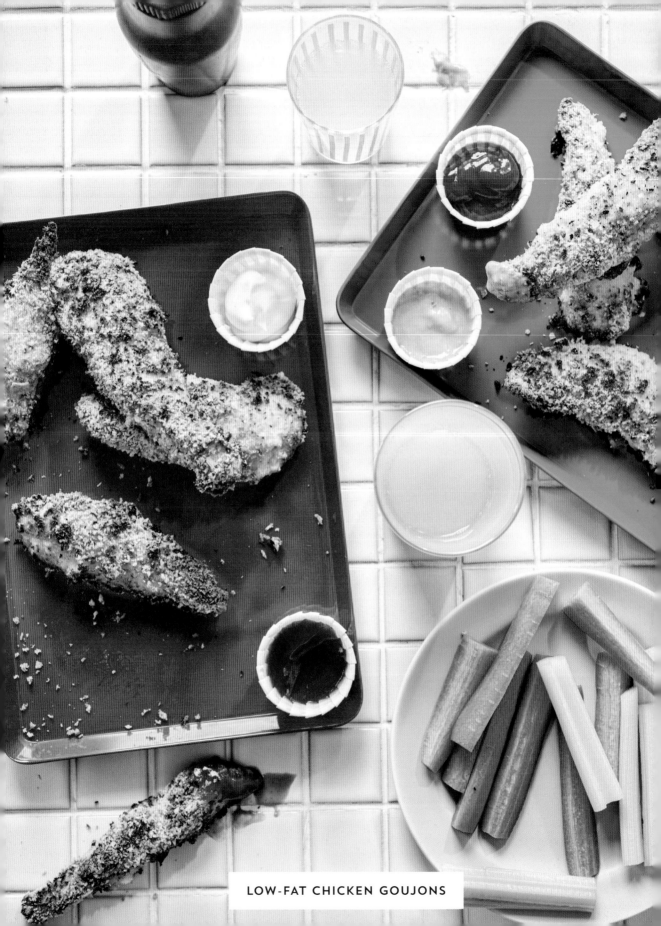

LOW-FAT CHICKEN GOUJONS

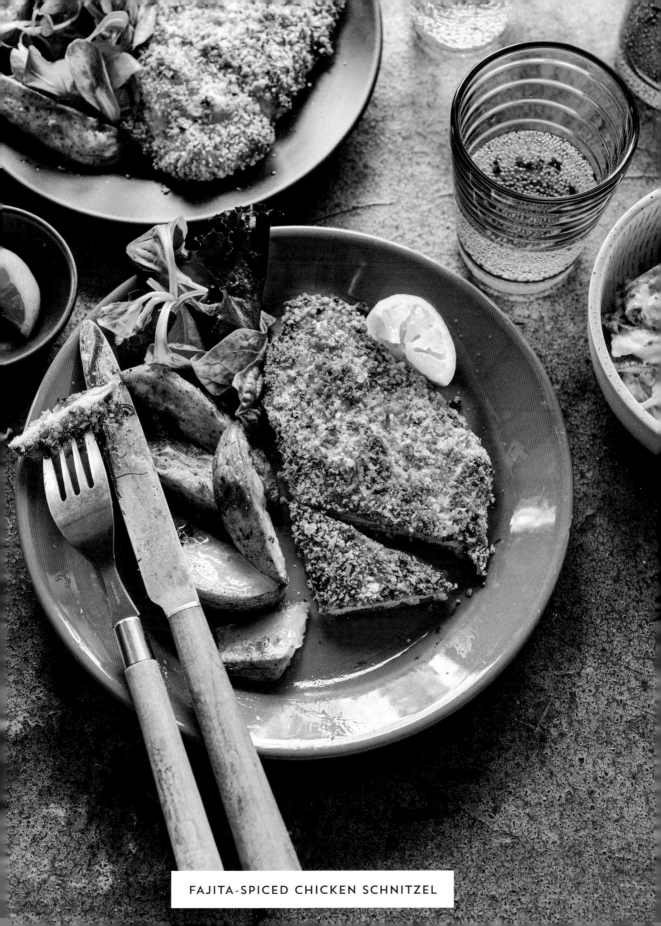

FAJITA-SPICED CHICKEN SCHNITZEL

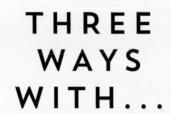

THREE WAYS WITH...

LOW-FAT CHICKEN GOUJONS

Now that you've prepared your Low-Fat Chicken Goujons, what are you going to do with them? Here are three simple ideas for different ways of serving them that will keep mealtimes feeling fresh and different every time. Each meal serves 4.

CHICKEN GOUJON PANINIS WITH SALAD & COLESLAW

1 x quantity Low-Fat Chicken
  Goujons (p.126)
8 tbsp shop-bought coleslaw
4 panini rolls, sliced
mixed salad leaves
4 slices low-fat cheese

1   Cook the Chicken Goujons as per the instructions on page 126.
2   Spread 2 tablespoons of coleslaw over the bottom half of each panini roll and top with mixed salad leaves.
3   Divide the goujons between the rolls, top with a slice of cheese and serve.

CHICKEN GOUJONS WITH PIRI-PIRI SWEET POTATO CHIPS & CORN ON THE COB

1 x quantity Piri-Piri Sweet Potato Chips (p.205)
1 x quantity Low-Fat Chicken Goujons (p.126)
4 x corn on the cob

1 Cook the Sweet Potato Chips as per the instructions on page 205.
2 Meanwhile, cook the Chicken Goujons as per the instructions on page 126.
3 5 minutes before the chips and goujons have finished cooking, add the corn on the cob to a large pan of boiling water over a medium heat. Cook for 5 minutes, until tender, then drain.
4 Serve the goujons with the chips and corn on the cob alongside.

CHICKEN GOUJONS CAESAR SALAD

1 x quantity Low-Fat Chicken Goujons (p.126)
1 x quantity Low-Fat Caesar Dressing (p.211)
1 head Cos lettuce, leaves stripped and washed
1 handful shop-bought croutons

1 Cook the Chicken Goujons as per the instructions on page 126.
2 While the goujons are cooking, make the Caesar Dressing as per the instructions on page 211.
3 Shred the lettuce leaves and put in a large bowl, then add the dressing and toss to combine.
4 Divide the salad between 4 serving bowls and top with the chicken goujons and a scattering of croutons. Serve.

ASPARAGUS-STUFFED CHICKEN WITH PROSCIUTTO

PREP: 10–15 MINS **COOK:** 25–30 MINS **SERVES:** 4 **SUGAR:** 3G **KCAL:** 253

This is the homemade equivalent of one of those fancy (and expensive) ready-prepped chicken ready-meals that comes in a foil tray that you can just stick in the oven and forget about, but it has the benefit of being both healthier and far kinder on the purse strings.

4 skinless, boneless chicken
  breasts
4 tbsp low-fat cream cheese
8 asparagus tips
8 slices prosciutto
salt and freshly ground pepper

To serve
Lighter Serve: Big leafy salad and your choice of dressing (p.210–11)
Family Serve: Mashed potatoes and veg of your choice

1   Place a chicken breast flat on a chopping board and press down with the palm of your hand. Working from the thickest end of the breast, insert a sharp knife two-thirds of the way through the meat and carefully slice down the length to the thinnest end to create a pocket. Repeat with the remaining chicken breasts.

> *If you are also making the Turkey-Wrapped Leek-And-Cheese-Stuffed Chicken, prep the chicken breasts for both dishes at the same time.*

2   Spoon a tablespoon of the cream cheese into the pocket of each chicken breast and top with 2 asparagus tips. Close the chicken breasts over the filling and wrap each one with 2 slices of prosciutto, then season with salt and pepper.

TO COOK
Transfer to a foil-lined baking tray and cook in an oven preheated to 180°C/350°F/gas mark 4 for 25–30 minutes, until cooked through, tender and juicy.

TO FREEZE
Transfer the uncooked, stuffed chicken breasts to a labelled freezer bag and freeze flat for up to 3 months.

TO COOK FROM FROZEN
Remove the stuffed chicken breasts for the freezer and leave to defrost fully in the fridge, ideally overnight, then cook as described in the *To Cook* section, left, ensuring the chicken is piping hot all the way through before serving.

TURKEY-WRAPPED LEEK-AND-CHEESE-STUFFED CHICKEN

PREP: 10–15 MINS **COOK:** 35 MINS **SERVES:** 4 **SUGAR:** 3G **KCAL:** 284

Another great stuffed chicken breast recipe that can be made ahead and kept in the freezer for an easy supper that can be on the table quickly but feels special enough to serve to guests. Prepping these is the work of moments, so why not double-up and make a big batch for the freezer?

4 skinless, boneless chicken
  breasts
1 small leek, finely chopped
3 tbsp low-fat cream cheese
½ cup (30g) low-fat, pre-grated
  cheddar cheese
8 rashers turkey bacon
salt and freshly ground pepper

To serve
Lighter Serve: Sliced into a salad
or served with seasonal vegetables
Family Serve: New potatoes and
seasonal vegetables

1 Place a chicken breast flat on a chopping board and press down with the palm of your hand. Working from the thickest end of the breast, insert a sharp knife two-thirds of the way through the meat and carefully slice down the length to the thinnest end to create a pocket. Repeat with the remaining chicken breasts.
2 Put the chopped leek, cream cheese, cheddar cheese and a grinding of salt and pepper in a small bowl and stir to combine.
3 Spoon a tablespoon of the leek and cheese mixture into the pocket of each chicken breast, then wrap each breast with 2 slices of turkey bacon, using a couple of cocktail sticks to secure the bacon, if necessary.

TO COOK

Lay the stuffed chicken breasts on a foil-lined baking tray, then transfer to an oven preheated to 180°C/350°F/gas mark 4 for 30–35 minutes, until cooked through, tender and juicy. Serve hot with your choice of sides.

TO FREEZE

Transfer the uncooked stuffed chicken breasts to a large, labelled freezer bag and freeze flat for up to 3 months.

TO COOK FROM FROZEN

Remove the stuffed chicken breasts for the freezer and leave to defrost fully in the fridge, ideally overnight, then cook as described in the *To Cook* section, left, ensuring the chicken is piping hot all the way through before serving.

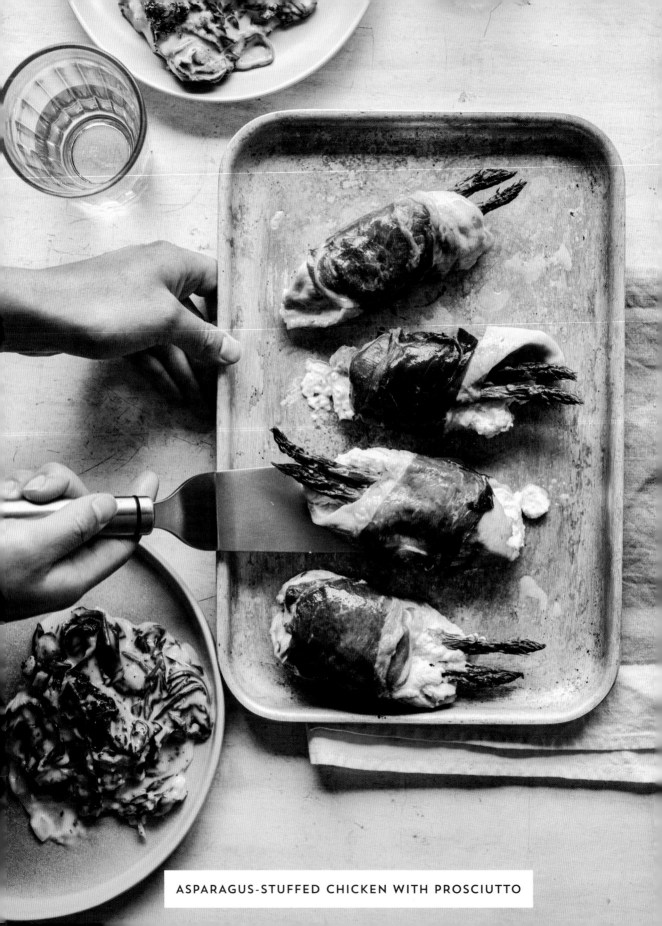

ASPARAGUS-STUFFED CHICKEN WITH PROSCIUTTO

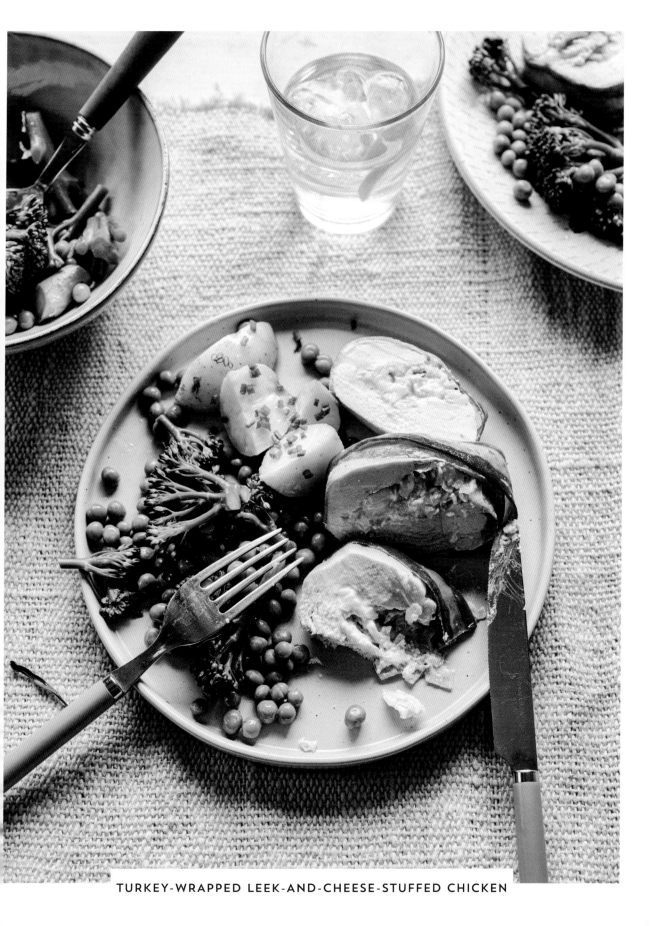

TURKEY-WRAPPED LEEK-AND-CHEESE-STUFFED CHICKEN

SPICED CAULIFLOWER STEAKS

PREP: 10 MINS **COOK:** 20–25 MINS **SERVES:** 4 **SUGAR:** 4.3G **KCAL:** 206

There make a wonderful meat-free alternative for burger nights and can easily be dressed up with all your favourite toppings and sauces. They can also be cooked straight from the freezer, so are a great fuss-free midweek option when you want an easy-win supper on the table in a flash. Feel free to play with the spices used in the coating and adapt them to the tastes of you and your family.

1 large cauliflower, leaves removed
1 tsp ground cumin
1 tsp paprika
1 tsp garlic powder
½ cup (55g) plain flour
3 eggs
1 cup (45g) panko breadcrumbs
low-calorie cooking spray
salt and freshly ground pepper

To serve
Lighter Serve: On half a burger bun with salad and sriracha sauce
Family Serve: In a burger bun, topped with cheese and with Piri-Piri Sweet Potato Chips (p.205) alongside

1 Put the cauliflower, stalk-end down, on a chopping board. Using a sharp knife, trim the ends off two sides of the cauliflower, leaving a flat edge on each, then slice the cauliflower into 1cm (½in) steaks. You will need 4.

> If you are also making the Harissa Cauliflower Traybake, add any remaining cauliflower from the steaks to the mix before baking. If not, simply transfer any remaining cauliflower to a labelled bag and freeze for a later date.

2 Put the cumin, paprika, garlic powder and flour in a shallow bowl and stir briefly to combine. Crack the eggs into a second bowl and beat with a fork. Put the panko breadcrumbs in a third bowl and season with a generous grinding of salt and pepper, then set all 3 bowls next to each other on the worktop.

3 Working with one steak at a time, dredge the cauliflower in the flour, shaking off any excess, then dip in the egg and, finally, press into the panko breadcrumbs until well coated on all sides. Repeat with the remaining steaks.

TO COOK

Lay the cauliflower steaks on a baking parchment-lined baking tray and spray each one with some low-calorie cooking spray, then transfer to an oven preheated to 180°C/350°F/gas mark 4 for 20–25 minutes, until the cauliflower is tender and the coating is golden and crunchy.

TO FREEZE

Transfer the uncooked coated cauliflower steaks to a large, labelled freezer bag in a single layer and freeze flat for up to 3 months.

TO COOK FROM FROZEN

These can be cooked directly from frozen. Lay the frozen, coated cauliflower steaks on a baking parchment-lined baking tray and spray each one with low-calorie cooking spray. Transfer to an oven preheated to 180°C/350°F/gas mark 4 and cook for 25–30 minutes, until golden brown and piping hot all of the way through.

HARISSA CAULIFLOWER TRAYBAKE

PREP: 10 MINS **COOK:** 30 MINS **SERVES:** 4 **SUGAR:** 11G **KCAL:** 289

This is a great one-pan, vegetarian meal that takes only moments to assemble and is kind on the wallet. The harissa packs a bit of a punch, so use as much or as little as you like to suit the tastes of your family.

2 cups (200g) cauliflower florets
2 cups (350g) fresh sliced mixed
  peppers
2 red onions, roughly chopped
1 x 400g can chickpeas, drained
2 tsp frozen chopped garlic
2–3 tsp harissa paste, to taste
3 tbsp olive oil
salt and freshly ground pepper
For the Harissa Sauce
  (make on day of serving):
½ cup (110g) low-fat natural
  yoghurt
1 tsp harissa paste
juice of 1 lemon

To serve

Lighter Serve: In a low-fat tortilla wrap with low-fat feta and the Harissa Sauce spooned over
Family Serve: With couscous, feta cheese and the Harissa Sauce spooned over

1 Put the cauliflower, peppers, onions, drained chickpeas, garlic, harissa paste and oil in a large bowl and mix well to ensure everything is well coated.

TO COOK

Pour the cauliflower mixture into a large baking dish and cook in an oven preheated to 180°C/350°F/ gas mark 4 for 30 minutes, until the veg is tender and golden. While the dish is in the oven, combine all of the sauce ingredients in a small bowl and stir well to combine. Serve the traybake with the sauce alongside for spooning over.

TO FREEZE

Transfer the uncooked cauliflower mixture to a large, labelled freezer bag and freeze flat for up to 3 months.

TO COOK FROM FROZEN

This can be defrosted and cooked as described left, or cooked from frozen by breaking the contents of the freezer bag into a baking dish and cooking at 180°C/350°F/gas mark 4 for 40 minutes, until piping hot. Either way, combine all of the ingredients for the sauce while the traybake is cooking and serve alongside for spooning.

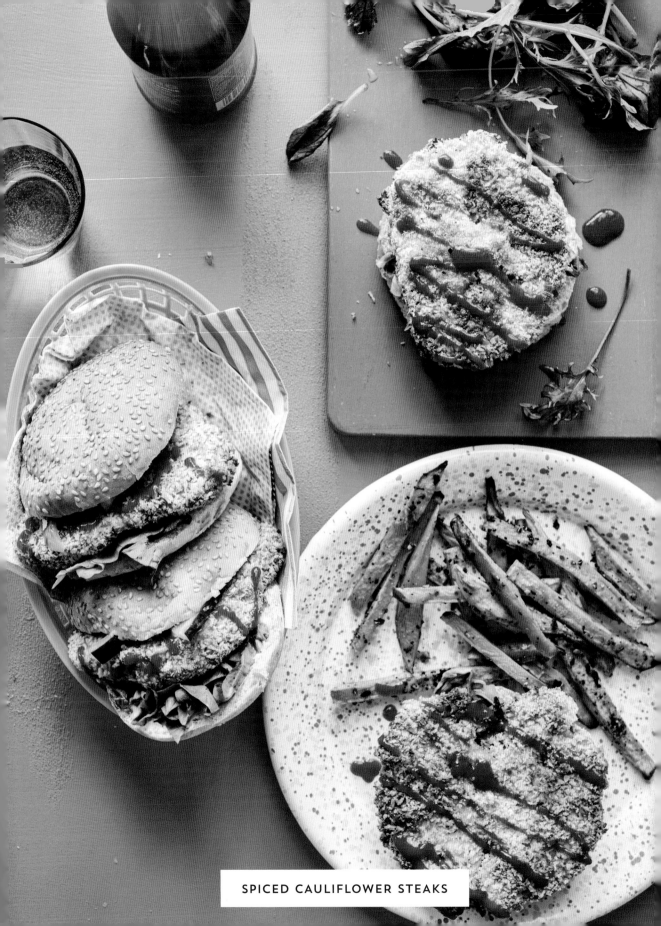

SPICED CAULIFLOWER STEAKS

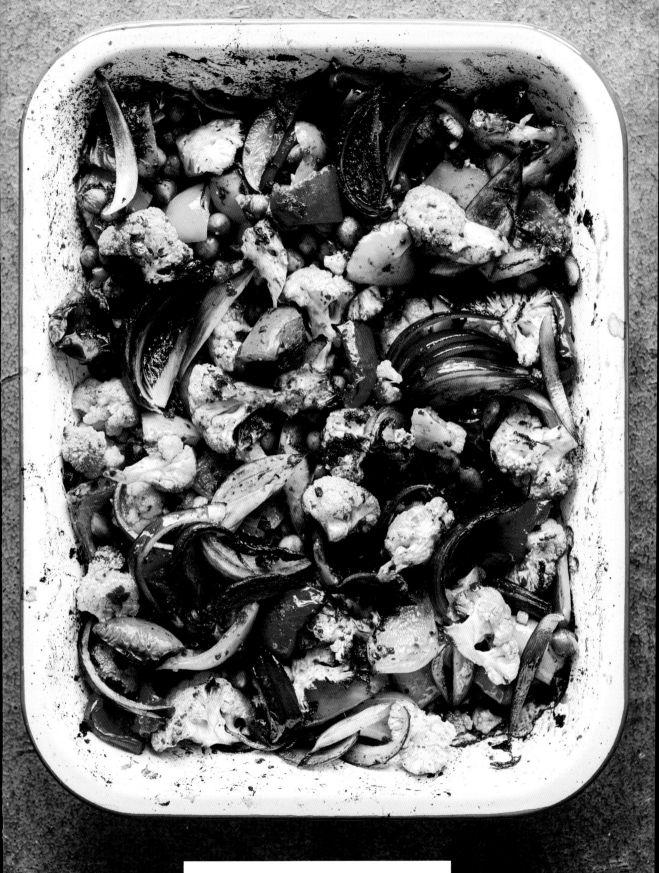

HARISSA CAULIFLOWER TRAYBAKE

TURKEY 'SHEPHERD'S' PIE

PREP: 10 MINS **COOK:** 1 HR 10 MINS **SERVES:** 6 **SUGAR:** 9.4G **KCAL:** 506

Turkey is a much leaner alternative to lamb, and this lighter version of a much-loved family classic always goes down a treat in my house. For ease, I have used shop-bought mashed potatoes in this recipe, but for an even lighter dish, feel free to substitute this with the Low-Cal Cheesy Mash recipe on page 202 of this book.

1 tbsp olive oil

1 cup (115g) frozen chopped onions

1 tsp frozen chopped garlic

500g lean turkey mince

1 heaped tbsp plain flour

1 cup (70g) grated carrot

1 cup (70g) mushrooms, chopped

2 tbsp tomato purée

2 cups (480ml) low-sodium chicken stock

1 tsp dried rosemary

2 tbsp Worcestershire sauce

2 x 425g packs pre-cooked mashed potatoes

1 cup (60g) low-fat, pre-grated cheddar cheese (optional)

To serve
Lighter Serve: Steamed green veg
Family Serve: Crusty French bread and your choice of vegetables

1   Heat the oil in a large saucepan over a medium heat. Add the onions and garlic and cook, stirring, for about 2 minutes, until soft.
2   Add the turkey mince, breaking it up with a wooden spoon, and cook, stirring regularly, until browned.
3   Add the flour, carrot, mushrooms, tomato purée, chicken stock, dried rosemary and Worcestershire sauce and stir to combine. Bring the mixture to the boil, then reduce the heat to a gentle simmer and leave to cook for 25 minutes, stirring occasionally, until the mixture has thickened and the turkey mince is cooked through.

> If you are also making the Spicy Turkey Burgers, assemble them now while the pie filling is cooking.

4   Once the pie filling has thickened, remove the pan from the heat and pour the mixture into a large baking dish.
5   Crumble the pre-made mash over the top of the pie filling in an even layer and sprinkle over the grated cheese, if using.

TO COOK

Transfer the pie to an oven preheated to 180°C/350°F/gas mark 4 for 30 minutes until the filling is bubbling and the top is golden. Serve hot with your choice of accompaniments.

TO FREEZE

Set the pie aside to cool to room temperature, then either cover with a lid or a layer of foil followed by a layer of clingfilm, label and freeze for up to 3 months.

TO COOK FROM FROZEN

This can be cooked straight from the freezer. Uncover the pie and transfer to an oven preheated to 180°C/350°F/gas mark 4 for 1 hour 10 minutes, until piping hot throughout. Cover with foil if the top starts to catch.

SPICY TURKEY BURGERS

PREP: 10 MINS **COOK:** 12–16 MINS **MAKES:** 8 BURGERS **SUGAR:** 0.5G **KCAL:** 216

Trying to eat healthily needn't mean missing out on the things you love and, whether served in a bun with wedges on the side or just with a simple salad, these spicy burgers will satisfy all of your burger cravings without any of the guilt! If you are making these for kids, feel free to play with the spices (or cut them out entirely) to suit their tastes.

1 small red onion, finely chopped
500g lean turkey mince
1 tsp paprika
1 tsp cayenne pepper
½ cup (25g) panko breadcrumbs
1 egg, beaten
salt and freshly ground pepper

To serve

Lighter Serve: On half a burger bun with salad on the side
Family Serve: In a burger bun with salad and with Skin-On Chips (p.204) or Piri-Piri Sweet Potato Chips (p.205) alongside

1 Line a baking tray with greaseproof paper.
2 Put all the ingredients in a large mixing bowl and season with a generous grinding of salt and pepper. Using your hands, bring the mixture together until everything is well combined. Still using your hands, form the mixture into 8 equal-sized balls and press each one down into a patty, then set aside on the prepared baking tray.

Make it Veggie!

For a vegetarian version, substitute the turkey mince with fresh, plant-based mince and make the burgers in the same way. If you struggle to form the balls, add an extra egg to help bind the mixture.

TO COOK

Lay the burgers on a grill pan and preheat the grill to high. Once the grill is hot, place the burgers under the heat and cook for 6–8 minutes on each side, until cooked through.

TO FREEZE

Cut 8 squares of greaseproof paper, each one slightly larger than the size of a burger and place a raw burger on each – this will prevent the burgers from sticking together and will allow you to remove them from the freezer individually. Stack the burgers on top of each other and transfer to a labelled freezer bag. Freeze for up to 3 months.

TO COOK FROM FROZEN

The burgers can be defrosted in the fridge overnight before cooking or cooked from frozen. If cooking from defrosted, follow the instructions in the *To Cook* section, left. If cooking from frozen, cook the burgers under the grill in the same way but increase the cooking time to 10–12 minutes on each side and ensure they are piping hot all the way through before serving.

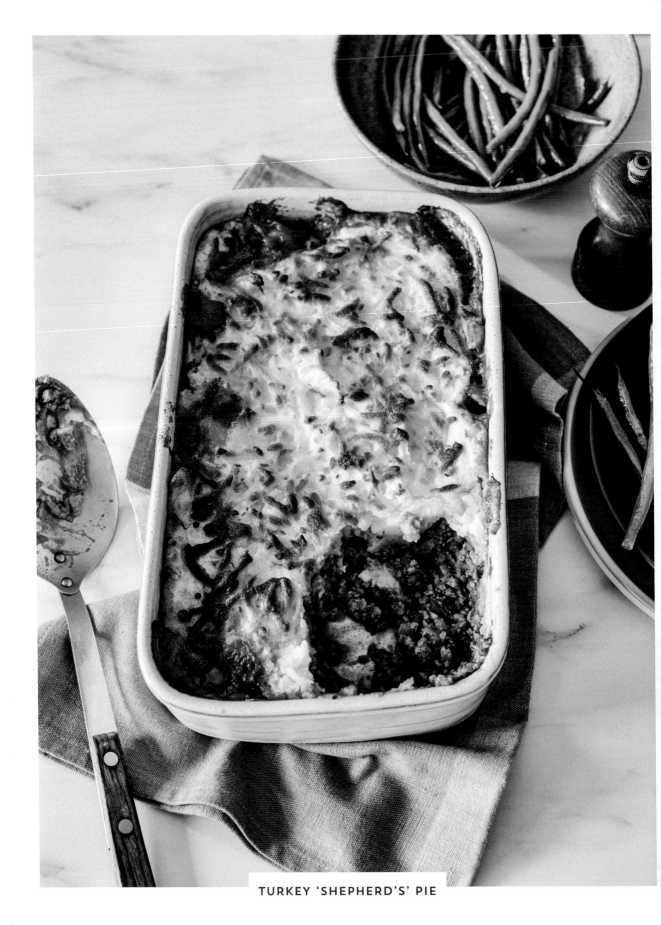

TURKEY 'SHEPHERD'S' PIE

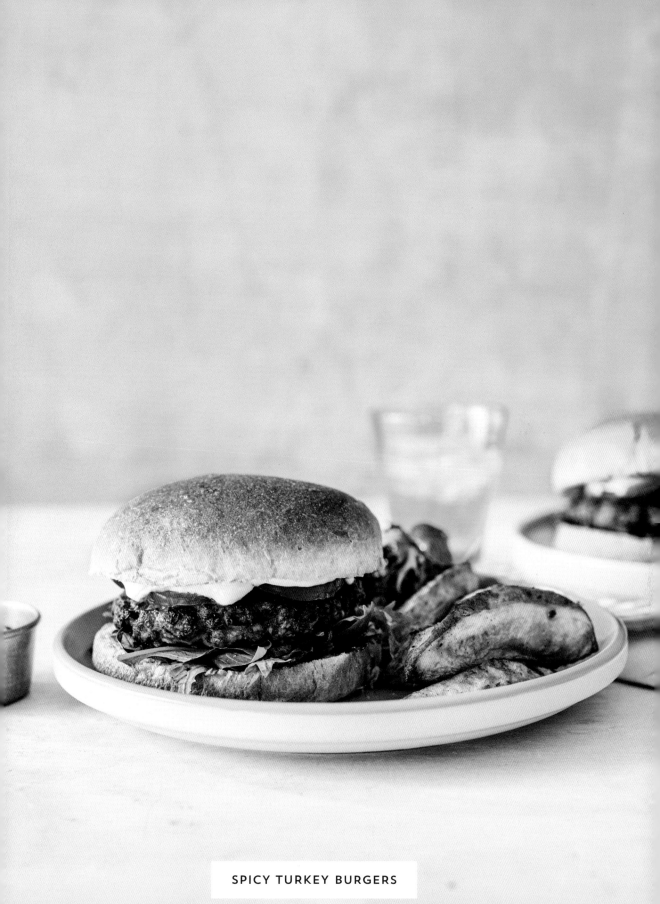

SPICY TURKEY BURGERS

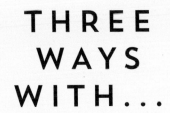

THREE WAYS WITH...

SPICY TURKEY BURGERS

Now that you've prepared your Spicy Turkey Burgers, what are you going to do with them? Here are three simple ideas for different ways of serving them that will keep mealtimes feeling fresh and different every time. Each meal serves 4.

TURKEY BURGERS WITH BAKED POTATOES & VEGGIES

4 baking potatoes
1 x quantity Spicy Turkey Burgers
  (p.141)
2 cups (300g) frozen mixed
  vegetables

1 Preheat the oven to 180°C/350°F/gas mark 4. Prick the potatoes all over with a fork and place on a foil-lined baking tray. Transfer to the oven to cook for 1 hour, until crisp on the outside and tender on the inside.

2 While the potatoes are cooking, cook the Spicy Turkey Burgers as per the instructions on page 141.

3 10 minutes before the potatoes and burgers are ready to serve, bring a pan of water to the boil. Add the frozen vegetables, reduce the heat to a gentle simmer and cook for 5 minutes, until tender. Drain through a colander.

4 Serve the burgers with the baked potatoes and cooked vegetables alongside.

SPICY TURKEY BURGER SALAD WITH MOZZARELLA

1 x quantity Spicy Turkey Burgers (p.141)

large bowl of mixed salad of your choice (I like salad leaves, sweetcorn, chopped boiled eggs, sliced cucumber, chopped tomatoes and sliced avocado)

1 x 125g ball low-fat mozzarella, drained

1 Cook the Spicy Turkey Burgers as per the instructions on page 141.
2 Divide the salad between 4 serving bowls.
3 Once cooked, cut the burgers into 2.5cm (1in) squares and scatter over the salad.
4 Rip the mozzarella into bite-sized chunks, scatter over the salad and serve.

TURKEY BURGERS, PITTA BREAD & HUMMUS

1 x quantity Spicy Turkey Burgers (p.141)

4 wholemeal pitta breads

1 small tub shop-bought hummus

1 pack mixed salad leaves

1 Cook the Spicy Turkey Burgers as per the instructions on page 141.
2 Toast the pitta breads briefly, then carefully split them open.
3 Once cooked, slice the burgers into 2.5cm (1in) strips, then stuff the pittas with the hummus, salad leaves and burger slices. Serve.

WHITE TURKEY CHILLI

PREP: 10 MINS **COOK:** 35–40 MINS **SERVES:** 4 **SUGAR:** 5.7G **KCAL:** 344

1 tbsp olive oil

1 cup (115g) frozen chopped onions

1 tsp frozen chopped garlic

500g lean turkey mince

2 tbsp plain flour

2 tsp ground cumin

1 tsp ground coriander

1 tsp chilli powder (optional)

1 cup (175g) frozen mixed peppers

2 cups (480ml) low-sodium chicken stock

½ cup (80g) canned or frozen sweetcorn (drained if canned)

½ cup (95g) canned red kidney beans, drained

1 tbsp low-fat crème fraiche

To serve

Lighter Serve: Over Cauliflower Rice (p.203) with fresh coriander sprinkled over

Family Serve: Over brown rice with a spoonful of natural yoghurt and fresh coriander sprinkled over

1. Heat the oil in a large saucepan over a medium heat. Add the onions and garlic and cook, stirring, for about 2 minutes, until soft.
2. Add the turkey mince, breaking it up with a wooden spoon, and cook, stirring regularly, until browned.
3. Add the flour and spices to the pan and stir to combine, then add the peppers and chicken stock and stir again. Bring to the boil, then reduce the heat to a gentle simmer and leave to cook, stirring occasionally, for 25 minutes.

> If you are also making the Chipotle Turkey Meatballs, make these now while the chilli is cooking.

4. Once the chilli has thickened and reduced, add the sweetcorn and kidney beans, stir and leave to cook for a final 5 minutes. Stir the crème fraiche through the chilli and remove the pan from the heat.

Make it Veggie!

To make this suitable for vegetarians, swap the turkey mince with fresh or frozen plant-based mince and cook the chilli in the same way. Plant-based mince tends to cook quicker than meat, so adjust the cooking time according to packet instructions.

TO SERVE

The chilli is now ready to serve with your choice of accompaniments.

TO FREEZE

Leave the chilli to cool to room temperature, then transfer to a large, labelled freezer bag and freeze flat for up to 3 months.

TO REHEAT FROM FROZEN

This can be defrosted in the fridge overnight and then reheated in a pan until piping hot, or cooked from frozen. If cooking from frozen, tip the chilli into a large pan, cover with a lid and place over a low heat. Cook, removing the lid occasionally and breaking it up with a spoon as the mixture defrosts, until it is fully defrosted and piping hot all of the way through.

CHIPOTLE TURKEY MEATBALLS

PREP: 10 MINS **COOK:** 15-20 MINS **SERVES:** 4 **SUGAR:** 0.5G **KCAL:** 215

500g lean turkey mince
½ tsp chipotle paste
1 tsp ground cumin
1 tsp smoked paprika
½ cup (25g) panko breadcrumbs
1 egg, beaten
salt and freshly ground pepper

To serve

Lighter Serve: In wholemeal pitta breads with salad and hummus
Family Serve: On wholewheat pasta topped with Smoky Sauce (p.219) and grated cheese

1 Line a baking tray with greaseproof paper.
2 Put all the ingredients in a large mixing bowl and season with a generous grinding of salt and pepper. Using your hands, bring the mixture together until everything is well combined, then form the mixture into 12 equal-sized balls, each just smaller than a golf ball, and set aside on the prepared baking tray.

Make it Veggie!

For a vegetarian version, substitute the turkey mince with fresh, plant-based mince and make the meatballs in the same way. If you struggle to form the balls, add an extra egg to help bind the mixture.

TO COOK

Transfer the baking tray with the meatballs to an oven preheated to 180°C/350°F/gas mark 4 for 15–20 minutes, until cooked through. Serve hot with your choice of accompaniments.

TO FREEZE

Transfer the uncooked meatballs to a large, labelled freezer bag in a single layer and freeze for up to 3 months.

TO COOK FROM FROZEN

These can be cooked from frozen or defrosted in the fridge overnight and cooked as described, left. If cooking from frozen, remove the meatballs from the freezer and place on a greaseproof paper-lined baking tray, then place in an oven preheated to 160°C/300°F/gas mark 3 for 15 minutes. Turn the meatballs and increase the oven temperature to 180°C/350°F/gas mark 4 and cook for a further 15 minutes, until piping hot all the way through. Serve hot with your choice of accompaniments.

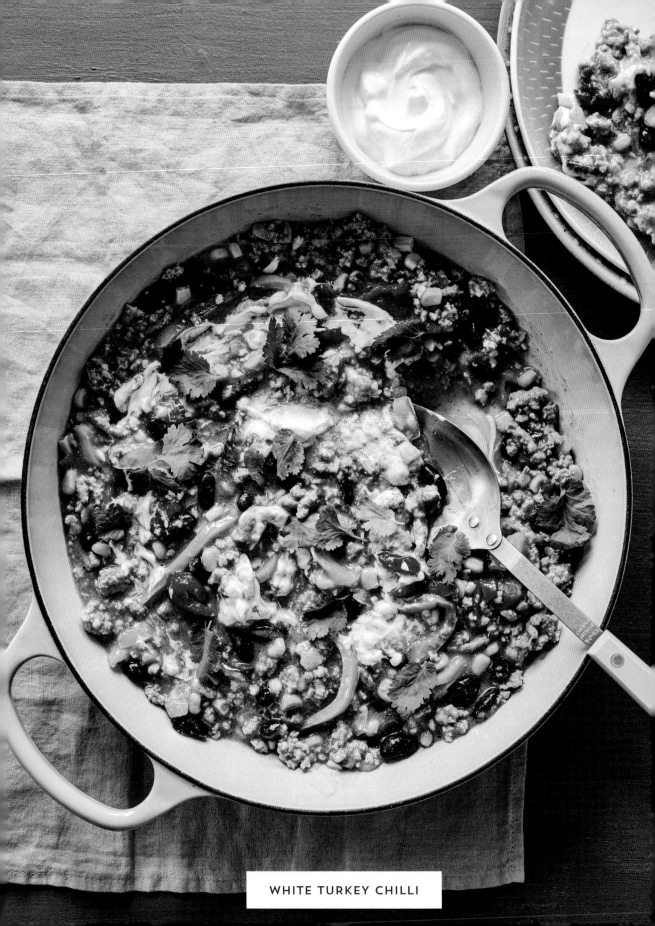

WHITE TURKEY CHILLI

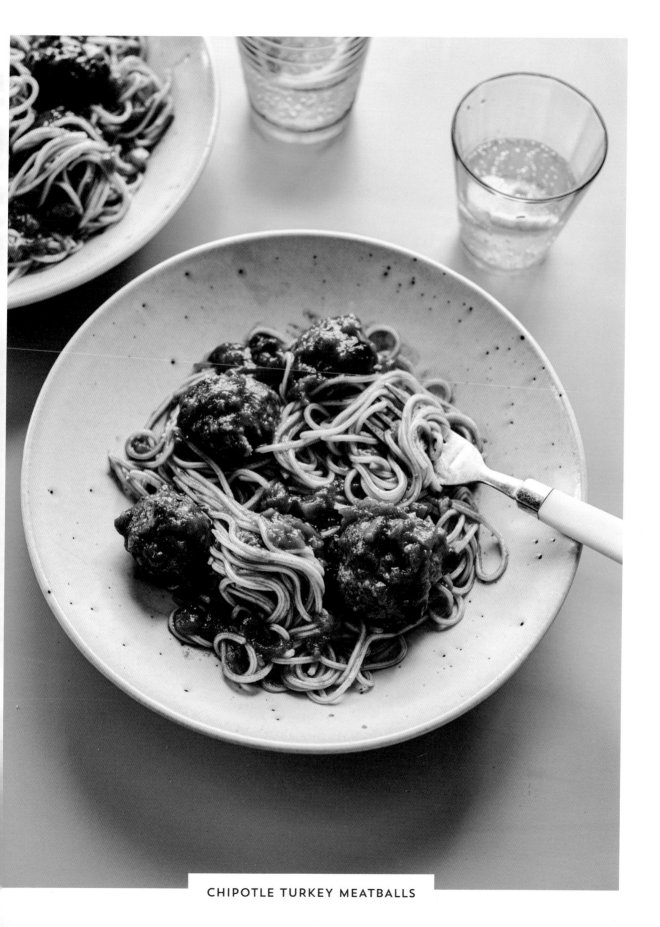

CHIPOTLE TURKEY MEATBALLS

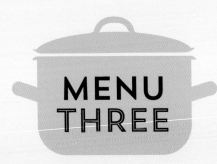

MENU THREE

3 FOR THE FRIDGE,
3 FOR THE FREEZER

Are you ready to batch three family meals for the week ahead and three to store in the freezer for another time in just 45 minutes? You will be making three recipes, each of which is doubled-up to feed eight people, so you simply need to split the recipe into two family meals before freezing one and putting the other in the fridge for the week ahead. The recipes are a mixture of cooked and no-cook freezer-bag meals, so while one recipe is bubbling away on the stove or cooking in the oven, you can be making the next meal ready for the fridge and freezer.

The shopping list on the opposite page includes everything you need and I have scaled up the ingredients for you so you don't need to worry about doubling the recipe. Simply buy what's on the shopping list and you will have everything you need to make the six meals. Once you have your shopping, lay the ingredients out into piles according to the groupings overleaf, so you have exactly what you need for each recipe to hand. Then simply follow the numbered guide and you can't go wrong!

Don't panic if this takes you more than 45 minutes the first time you cook it – you will get quicker each time you make it. So, roll up your sleeves, get cooking and think about the time you will be saving yourself in the future!

YOU WILL BE MAKING:

TURKEY BOLOGNESE
THAI CHICKEN NOODLE SOUP
LAMB MEATLOAF

SHOPPING LIST

Fresh

1kg lean turkey mince

1 x 200g pack pre-grated carrots

2 x 250g packs pre-sliced mushrooms

6 skinless, boneless chicken thighs

1kg lean lamb mince

2 limes

2 eggs

1 x 150g pack mange tout

Frozen

1 x 500g pack frozen chopped onions

1 x 75g pack frozen chopped garlic

1 x 75g pack frozen chopped ginger

1 x 50g pack frozen chopped parsley

Storecupboard

low-calorie cooking spray

1 tube tomato purée

1 jar dried oregano

1 x 285g jar Thai green curry paste

1 x 250ml bottle low-sodium soy sauce

2 tsp ground cumin

1 jar paprika

1 jar ground coriander

1 x 225g pack vermicelli noodles

2 x 400g cans reduced-fat coconut milk

4 x 400g cans chopped tomatoes

salt and pepper

4 low-sodium chicken stock cubes

olive oil

INGREDIENTS

GET ORGANISED! Before you start cooking, make sure that your kitchen surfaces are cleared down, then lay all the ingredients out in individual piles according to the groupings below.

TURKEY BOLOGNESE

low-calorie cooking spray
2 cups (230g) frozen chopped
  onions
2 tsp frozen chopped garlic
1kg lean turkey mince
2 cups (140g) pre-grated carrots
2 cups (140g) pre-sliced
  mushrooms
2 tbsp tomato purée
4 x 400g cans chopped tomatoes
2 cups (480ml) low-sodium
  chicken stock
1 tsp dried oregano
salt and freshly ground pepper

LAMB MEATLOAF

low-calorie cooking spray
2 cups (230g) frozen chopped
  onions
4 tsp frozen chopped garlic
1kg lean lamb mince
2 tsp ground cumin
2 tsp paprika
2 tsp ground coriander
2 tbsp tomato purée
4 tsp frozen chopped parsley
2 eggs, beaten
2 tsp salt
2 tbsp olive oil
freshly ground pepper

THAI CHICKEN NOODLE SOUP

7 cups (1.7lt) low-sodium chicken
  stock
2 x 400g cans reduced-fat
  coconut milk
4 tbsp Thai green curry paste, or
  to taste
4 tsp frozen chopped garlic
4 tsp frozen chopped ginger
6 skinless, boneless chicken thighs,
  cut into bite-sized pieces
2 tbsp low-sodium soy sauce
4 cups (280g) pre-sliced
  mushrooms
juice of 2 limes
On day of serving:
2 nests vermicelli noodles
1½ cups (130g) mange tout

METHOD

TURKEY BOLOGNESE

1 Spray a large saucepan with low-calorie cooking spray and place over a medium heat. Add the onions and garlic and cook, stirring continuously, for 2–3 minutes, until softened.

2 Add the turkey mince, breaking it up with a wooden spoon, and cook, stirring occasionally, for 10 minutes, until browned.

LAMB MEATLOAF

3 Spray a large saucepan with low-calorie cooking spray and place over a medium heat. Add the onions and garlic and cook, stirring continuously,

for 2–3 minutes, until softened. Remove from the heat and set aside.

THAI CHICKEN NOODLE SOUP

4 Place a large saucepan over a high heat and add the chicken stock, coconut milk, Thai curry paste, garlic and ginger and bring to the boil.

5 Once boiling, reduce the heat to a simmer and add the chicken, soy sauce, mushrooms and lime juice. Leave to cook for 8–10 minutes, stirring occasionally, until the chicken is cooked through.

TURKEY BOLOGNESE CONTINUED...

6 Once the turkey mince is browned, add in the grated carrots, sliced mushrooms, tomato purée, chopped tomatoes, chicken stock, dried oregano and a generous grinding of salt and pepper to the

pan and stir to combine. Leave to cook for around 25 minutes, until the sauce has thickened and reduced.

THAI CHICKEN NOODLE SOUP CONTINUED...

7 Once the chicken is cooked through, remove the soup from the heat and set aside to cool while you make your meatloaves.

CONTINUED OVERLEAF...

LAMB MEATLOAF CONTINUED...

8   Add the lamb mince, ground cumin, paprika, ground coriander, tomato purée, chopped parsley, beaten eggs, salt and a grinding of pepper to a large mixing bowl, then tip in the cooked onions and garlic from the frying pan. Using your hands, mix all of the ingredients together until really well combined.

9   Line 2 baking trays with foil and tip half of the lamb mixture onto each tray. Using your hands, shape each half of the mixture into a small loaf shape, roughly 15cm (6in) long x 7cm (2¾in) wide.

10 Cover 1 of the meatloaves with clingfilm and transfer to the fridge for the week ahead. Wrap the other meatloaf, still on the tray, in a layer of clingfilm and freeze for a couple of hours, until solid. Remove from the freezer and take the meatloaf off the baking tray, then rewrap it in a layer of foil, followed by a layer of clingfilm and freeze for up to 3 months.

TURKEY BOLOGNESE CONTINUED...

11 Once cooked, remove the bolognese from the heat and set aside to cool while you package up your soup.

THAI CHICKEN NOODLE SOUP CONTINUED...

12 Put half of the cooled soup into a large, labelled freezer bag (a zip-lock bag works best for this) and freeze flat for up to 3 months. Put the remaining soup in a container with a lid and keep in the fridge for the week ahead.

TURKEY BOLOGNESE CONTINUED...

13 Once cooled to room temperature, put half of the bolognese into a large, labelled freezer bag and freeze flat for up to 3 months. Put the remaining bolognese in a container with a lid and keep in the fridge for the week ahead.

Congratulations!

You have just made six meals!
Three for the week ahead
and three for the freezer.

WHEN YOU COME TO COOK

Once cooked, all of these meals are best fully defrosted before cooking. All reheated meals should reach a temperature of 74°C/165°F. Always make sure any reheated food is piping hot before serving. Cooking instructions for each dish are given below.

TURKEY BOLOGNESE

FROM THE FRIDGE

Pour the bolognese into a large pan and place over a medium heat until piping hot.

FROM THE FREEZER

Remove the bolognese from the freezer and leave to fully defrost in the fridge, ideally overnight. Once defrosted, transfer the bolognese to a large pan and place over a medium heat until piping hot.

To serve

Lighter Serve: On a bed of courgetti with a sprinkling of grated low-fat cheese
Family Serve: On a bed of wholewheat spaghetti with a sprinkling of grated Parmesan cheese and garlic bread on the side

THAI CHICKEN NOODLE SOUP

FROM THE FRIDGE

Pour the soup into a large pan and place over a medium heat until boiling, then reduce the heat to a simmer and add the vermicelli noodles and mange tout. Cook for another 3 minutes, until the noodles and veg are tender, then serve.

FROM THE FREEZER

Remove the soup from the freezer and leave to fully defrost in the fridge, ideally overnight. Once defrosted, pour the soup into a large pan and place over a medium heat until boiling, then reduce the heat to a simmer and add the vermicelli noodles and mange tout. Cook for another 3 minutes, until the noodles and veg are tender, then serve.

To serve

Lighter Serve: Wholemeal pitta breads
Family Serve: Crusty bread and butter

LAMB MEATLOAF

FROM THE FRIDGE

Preheat the oven to 160°C/300°F/gas mark 3. Remove the meatloaf from the fridge, remove the clingfilm and brush with 1 tablespoon of olive oil. Transfer to the oven for 50 minutes–1 hour, until cooked through. Cut into slices and serve.

FROM THE FREEZER

Remove the meatloaf from the freezer and leave to fully defrost in the fridge, ideally overnight. Once defrosted, preheat the oven to 160°C/300°F/gas mark 3. Remove the meatloaf from the fridge, remove the clingfilm and foil, and brush with 1 tablespoon of olive oil. Transfer to the oven for 50 minutes–1 hour, until cooked through. Cut into slices and serve.

To serve

Lighter Serve: Salad, Harissa Dressing (p.210)
Family Serve: Salad, Harissa Dressing (p.210) and Light-And-Easy Paprika Flatbreads (p.209)

WEEKEND
FEASTS

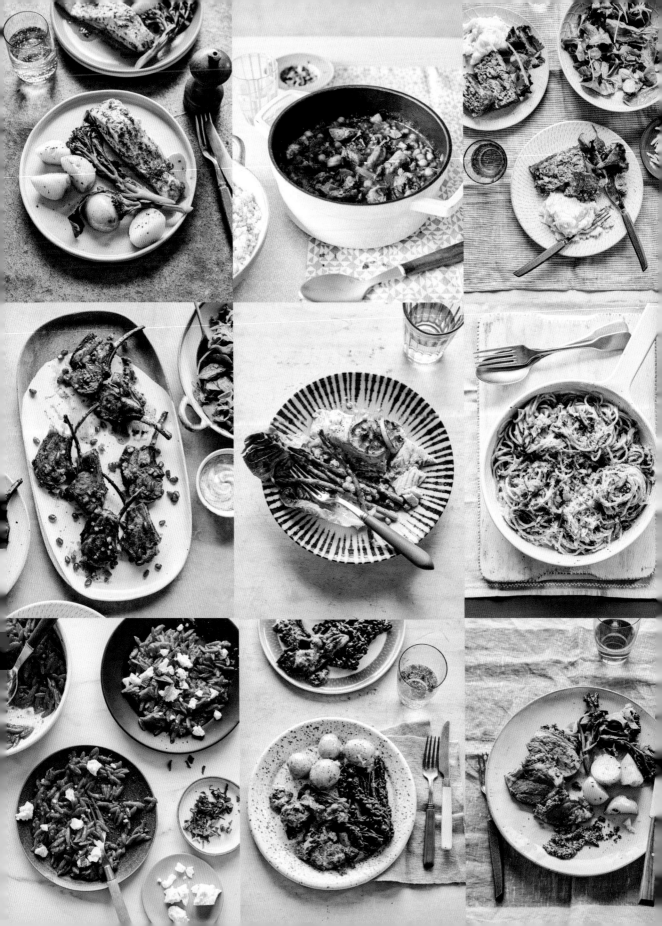

WEEKEND FEASTS

Spending a bit of time stirring a pot over a stove and preparing a meal for your loved ones can in itself be an act of self-care and, whether you're catering for a family meal or have guests for a dinner party, weekends are the pause in the week when we often have a little more time to make something that feels special. The recipes in this chapter aren't time-consuming, but you don't need to tell anybody that. Guests will believe you've spent hours stirring my creamy and delicious Sundried Tomato Risotto (p.183), for example, but in reality it is baked in the oven and couldn't be simpler.

The ingredients used here can be slightly more luxe than elsewhere, and fresh herbs and more expensive cuts of meat do come into play, such as in my Lamb Chops with Salsa Verde (p.179) or Herb-Crusted Lamb Rumps (p.161), but the main focus is on meals that will impress your family and guests with minimum effort on your behalf. For vegetarians, there is a stunning pink-hued Beetroot & Feta Orzotto (p.182) or a hearty, but surprisingly light, Mushroom Stroganoff (p.164).

A big pot of my Turkey Tagine (p.178) served in the middle of the table for everyone to dig in feels wonderfully celebratory and, for Sunday lunch, my Cajun Turkey-And-Pepper Meatloaf (p.175) makes a wonderful alternative to a traditional roast.

MOROCCAN-STYLE LAMB CHOPS

PREP: 5 MINS, PLUS MARINATING **COOK:** 10 MINS **SERVES:** 4 **SUGAR:** 0.5G **KCAL:** 351

These fragrant lamb chops make a wonderful centrepiece to a Middle Eastern-inspired banquet, but are just as special simply served with salad. I like to take these along to summer barbecues, where they are always a big hit with friends and family alike.

2 tbsp olive oil
1 tsp ground cumin
1 tsp ground coriander
1 tsp paprika
1 tsp frozen chopped garlic
juice of 1 lemon
1 tsp harissa paste
4 large (or 8 small) lamb chops
salt and freshly ground pepper

1 Combine the olive oil, cumin, coriander, paprika, garlic, lemon juice, harissa paste and a generous grinding of salt and pepper in a large bowl.
2 Tip the lamb chops into the bowl and massage the marinade into the meat with your hands, ensuring all of the chops are well coated. Set aside for 30 minutes to marinate.

> If you are also making the Herb-Crusted Lamb Rumps, assemble these now while the chops are marinating.

To serve
Lighter Serve: A big leafy salad and a scattering of fresh pomegranate seeds
Family Serve: Couscous, hummus, salad and Harissa Dressing (p.210)

TO COOK

Preheat the grill to high and line a grill pan with foil. Lay the marinated chops on the grill pan and place under the grill to cook for 3–4 minutes on each side, until cooked to your liking. Remove from the heat, cover with foil and leave to rest for 5 minutes before serving.

TO FREEZE

Transfer the uncooked marinated lamb chops to a large, labelled freezer bag in a single layer and freeze flat for up to 3 months.

TO COOK FROM FROZEN

Remove the lamb chops from the freezer and leave to defrost fully in the fridge, ideally overnight. Once defrosted, cook the lamb chops as described in the *To Cook* section, left.

HERB-CRUSTED LAMB RUMPS

PREP: 5-10 MINS **COOK:** 15-18 MINS, PLUS RESTING **SERVES:** 4 **SUGAR:** 1G **KCAL:** 337

This herb-crusted lamb dish makes a wonderful Sunday lunch and is far quicker and easier than cooking an entire joint in the oven. If you are trying to watch what you eat, then do trim the lamb fat to keep it nice and lean.

2 tsp dried thyme

2 tsp dried rosemary

1 tsp garlic granules

1 cup (45g) panko breadcrumbs

2 tbsp Dijon mustard

1 tsp frozen chopped parsley

4 lamb rump steaks, fat trimmed

salt and freshly ground pepper

To serve

Lighter Serve: Baked sweet potatoes and oven-roasted tomatoes

Family Serve: Boulangère Potatoes (p.199) and Carrots with Garlic & Tarragon (p.207)

1 Add the thyme, rosemary, garlic granules and breadcrumbs to a mini chopper or freestanding blender and pulse to a fine crumb.

2 Tip the crumbs into a bowl and add the mustard, parsley and a generous grinding of salt and pepper, then mix to combine.

3 Lay the lamb rump steaks on a chopping board and spoon the crust mixture over the top, dividing it equally between the steaks. Press the mixture down firmly to form a solid crust.

TO COOK

Transfer the lamb steaks to a foil-lined baking tray and cook in an oven preheated to 190°C/375°F/gas mark 5 for 15–18 minutes, until cooked to your liking. Remove from the oven and cover with foil, then leave to rest for 5 minutes before serving. Serve hot.

TO FREEZE

Transfer the crusted but uncooked lamb steaks to a large, labelled freezer bag in a single layer and freeze flat for up to 3 months.

TO COOK FROM FROZEN

Remove the lamb steaks from the freezer and leave to defrost in the fridge, ideally overnight. Once defrosted, cook the lamb steaks as described in the *To Cook* section, left.

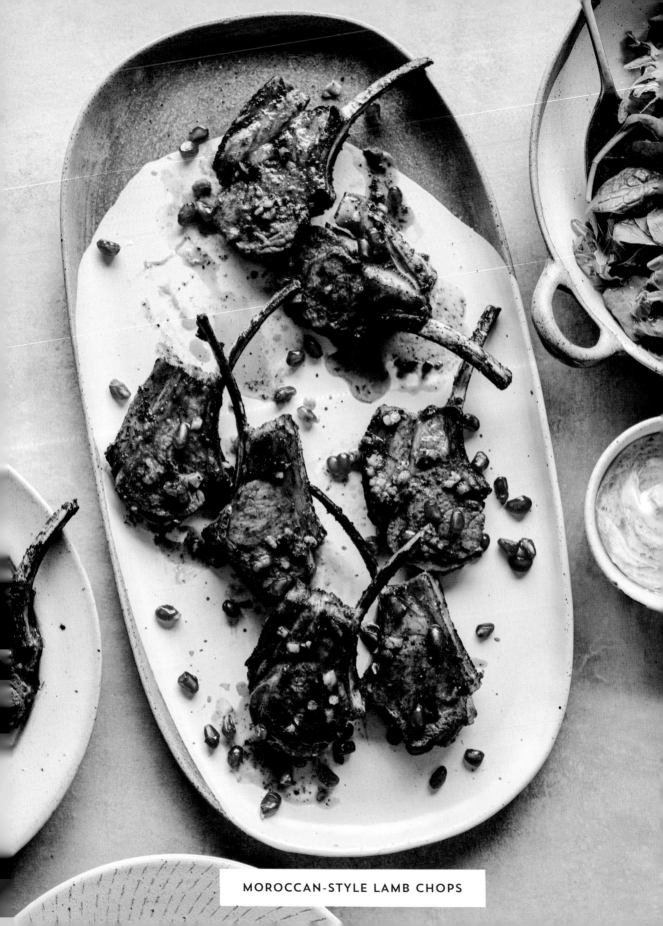

MOROCCAN-STYLE LAMB CHOPS

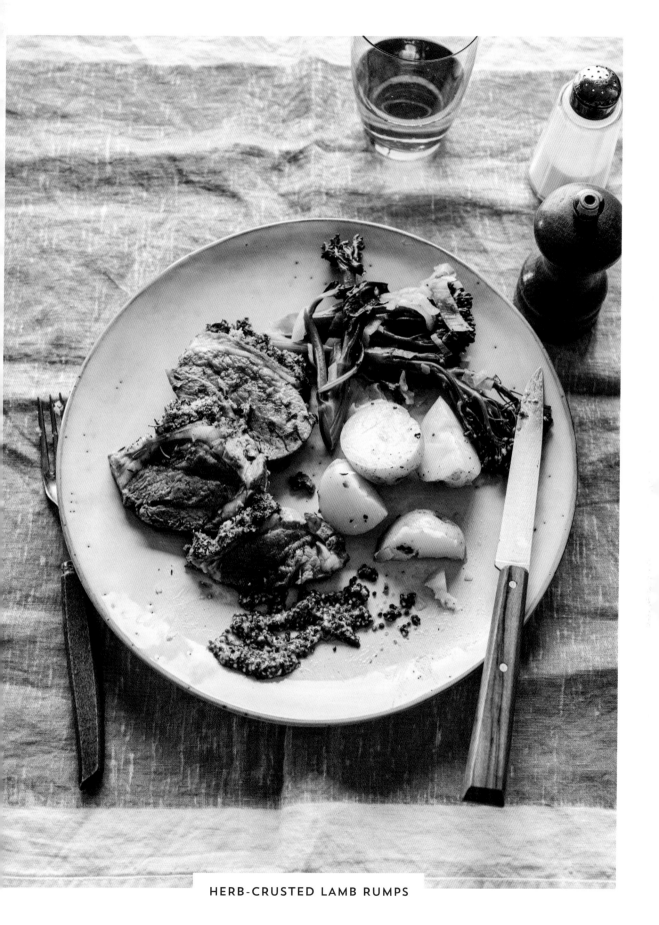

HERB-CRUSTED LAMB RUMPS

MUSHROOM STROGANOFF

PREP: 5 MINS **COOK:** 15–20 MINS **SERVES:** 4 **SUGAR:** 2.4G **KCAL:** 121

This warming stroganoff is so creamy and comforting that no-one will believe that it's low in fat. If making this for the freezer, make sure to omit the sour cream and add it just before serving as freezing it can cause it to split.

low-calorie cooking spray
1 cup (115g) frozen chopped onions
2 tsp frozen chopped garlic
600g white closed cup
   mushrooms, sliced
½ cup (120ml) low-sodium
   vegetable stock
1 tsp Dijon mustard
1 tsp frozen chopped parsley
salt and freshly ground pepper
1 cup (200g) low-fat sour cream
   to serve

To serve
Lighter Serve: Cauliflower Rice
(p.203) and green vegetables
Family Serve: Basmati rice and
green vegetables

1 Spray a large saucepan with low-calorie cooking spray and place over a medium heat. Add the onions and garlic and cook, stirring continuously, for 2–3 minutes, until soft.
2 Add the mushrooms and cook, stirring occasionally, for 6–8 minutes, until soft.

> If you are also making the Stuffed Portobello Mushrooms, assemble them now while the mushrooms for the stroganoff are cooking.

3 Add the vegetable stock, bring to the boil, then reduce the heat to a gentle simmer and cook, stirring occasionally, for 6 minutes, until slightly thickened.
4 Remove the pan from the heat and stir through the mustard and parsley.

TO SERVE

Stir the sour cream through the stroganoff and season to taste. Serve the stroganoff hot with your choice of accompaniments.

TO FREEZE

Leave the stroganoff to cool to room temperature, then transfer to a large, labelled freezer bag and freeze flat for up to 3 months.

TO REHEAT FROM FROZEN

This can be defrosted in the fridge overnight and then reheated in a pan until piping hot, or cooked from frozen. If cooking from frozen, tip the frozen stroganoff into a large saucepan, cover with a lid and place over a low heat. Cook, removing the lid occasionally and breaking it up with a wooden spoon as the mixture defrosts, until it is fully defrosted and piping hot all of the way through. Stir the sour cream through the stroganoff before serving.

STUFFED PORTOBELLO MUSHROOMS

PREP: 5 MINS **COOK:** 18-20 MINS **SERVES:** 4 **SUGAR:** 5.1G **KCAL:** 186

For the filling:

1 cup (200g) low-fat cream cheese

8 sundried tomatoes, drained and finely chopped

½ cup (40g) low-fat, pre-grated cheddar cheese

10 chives, finely chopped

1 handful fresh spinach, finely chopped

salt and freshly ground pepper

On day of serving:

4 portobello mushrooms

4 tsp panko breadcrumbs

low-calorie cooking spray

To serve

Lighter Serve: Rocket salad and your choice of dressing (p.210–11)

Family Serve: Buttered new potatoes, rocket salad and your choice of dressing (p.210–11)

1 Put all of the filling ingredients into a bowl with a grinding of salt and pepper and stir to combine.

TO COOK

Place the mushrooms on a foil-lined baking tray and divide the filling mixture between them, spooning it into the cups and pressing down to form an even layer. Sprinkle each mushroom with a teaspoon of panko breadcrumbs and spray each one a couple of times with low-calorie cooking spray. Transfer to an oven preheated to 180°C/350°F/gas mark 4 and cook for 18–20 minutes, until golden and tender.

TO FREEZE

Transfer the uncooked filling mixture to a labelled freezer bag and freeze flat for up to 3 months.

TO COOK FROM FROZEN

Remove the mushroom filling from the freezer and leave to fully defrost in the fridge, ideally overnight. Tip the mixture into a large bowl and stir to combine, then fill, dress and cook the mushrooms as described in the *To Cook* section, left.

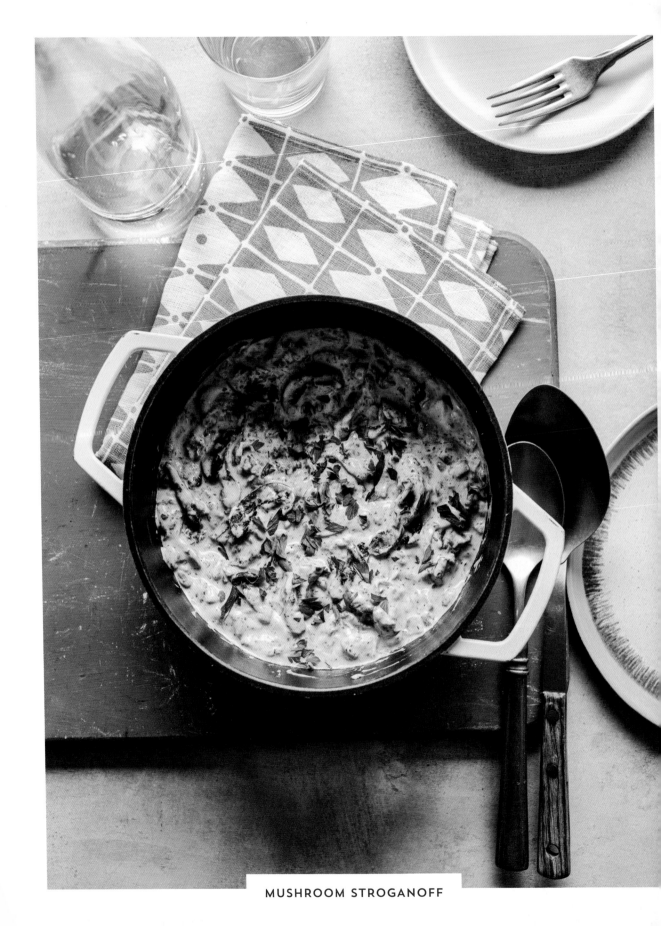

MUSHROOM STROGANOFF

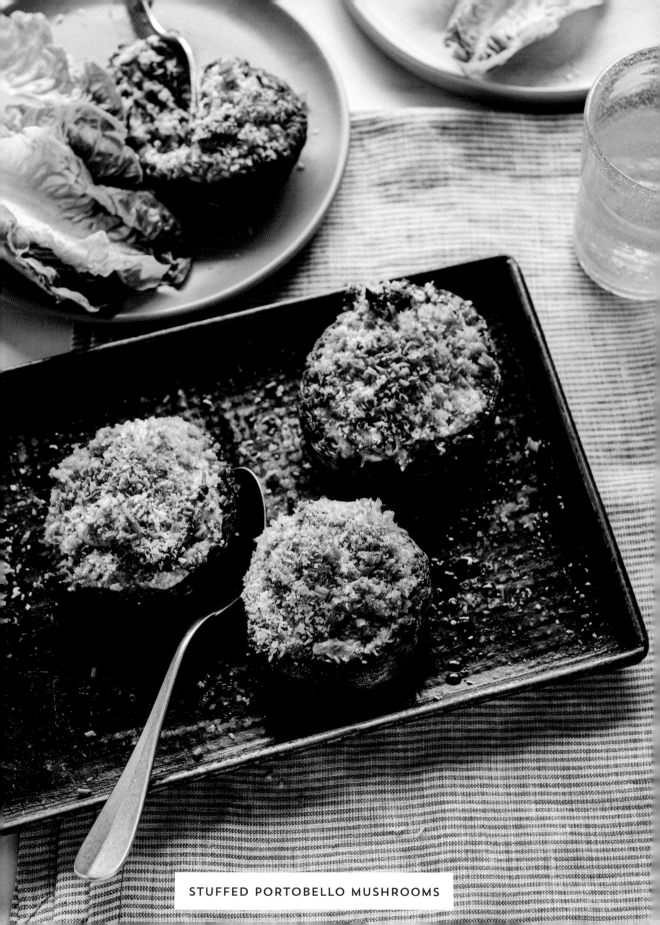

STUFFED PORTOBELLO MUSHROOMS

CREAMY SALMON & PEA PARCELS

PREP: 10 MINS **COOK:** 15–20 MINS **SERVES:** 4 **SUGAR:** 5.1G **KCAL:** 523

These dainty parcels of fish and peas make a great easy supper, as because they already contain a portion of healthy veg, they can be served as they are for a no-fuss meal that still feels weekend worthy. For bigger appetites, no one ever said no to a portion of chips on the side!

2 cups (310g) frozen peas
4 tbsp low-fat crème fraîche
2 tsp dried dill
4 salmon fillets
1 lemon, sliced
salt and freshly ground pepper

To serve
Lighter Serve: Cooked
wholewheat orzo
Family Serve: Skin-On Chips
(p.204)

1   Put the peas, crème fraîche, dill and a generous grinding of salt and pepper into a mixing bowl and stir to combine.
2   Lay 4 large sheets of foil side-by-side on the worktop and spoon a quarter of the pea and crème fraîche mixture into the centre of each one.
3   Lay a salmon fillet, skin-side down, on top of each mound of the pea and crème fraîche mixture and place a couple of slices of lemon on top of each salmon fillet.
4   Working with 1 sheet of foil at a time, bring up the sides to enclose the salmon and scrunch the edges together to form a parcel. Repeat until you have 4 parcels.

TO COOK

Lay the parcels on a baking tray and transfer to an oven preheated to 180°C/350°F/gas mark 4 for 15–20 minutes, until the salmon is cooked through. Serve hot with your choice of accompaniments.

TO FREEZE

Transfer the uncooked parcels to a large, labelled freezer bag and freeze flat for up to 3 months.

TO COOK FROM FROZEN

Remove the salmon parcels from the freezer and leave to defrost fully in the fridge, ideally overnight. Once defrosted, lay the parcels on a baking tray and transfer to an oven preheated to 180°C/350°F/ gas mark 4 for 15–20 minutes, until the salmon is cooked through.

CAJUN SALMON FILLETS

PREP: 5 MINS **COOK:** 15-18 MINS **SERVES:** 4 **SUGAR:** 0G **KCAL:** 390

Cajun seasoning adds a big punch of flavour to these super simple oven-baked salmon fillets.
If you are making this for the freezer, this really couldn't be simpler and can be bagged up and
ready to freeze in 5 minutes flat.

3 tsp Cajun seasoning
1 tsp dried thyme
2 tbsp olive oil
juice of 1 lemon
4 salmon fillets
salt and freshly ground pepper

To serve
Lighter Serve: New potatoes and
steamed green vegetables
Family Serve: Buttered new
potatoes and veg of your choice

1 Put the Cajun seasoning, dried thyme, olive oil, lemon juice and
a generous grinding of salt and pepper into a small bowl and stir
to combine.

TO COOK

Place a large sheet of foil on the
work surface and lay the salmon
fillets in the centre, skin-side down.
Pour over the marinade, ensuring
all of the salmon fillets are well
coated, then bring up the sides of
the foil to enclose the salmon and
scrunch it together to seal. Transfer
the foil parcel to a baking tray,
then cook in an oven preheated
to 180°C/350°F/gas mark 4 for
15–18 minutes, until the salmon
is cooked through. Serve hot with
your choice of accompaniments.

TO FREEZE

Transfer the uncooked salmon
fillets to a large, labelled freezer
bag and pour the marinade over the
top, massaging the sides of the bag
to ensure the salmon is well coated.
Seal the bag and freeze flat for up
to 3 months.

TO COOK FROM FROZEN

Remove the salmon from the
freezer and leave to defrost in the
fridge, ideally overnight. Once
defrosted, cook the salmon in a foil
parcel as described in the *To Cook*
section, left.

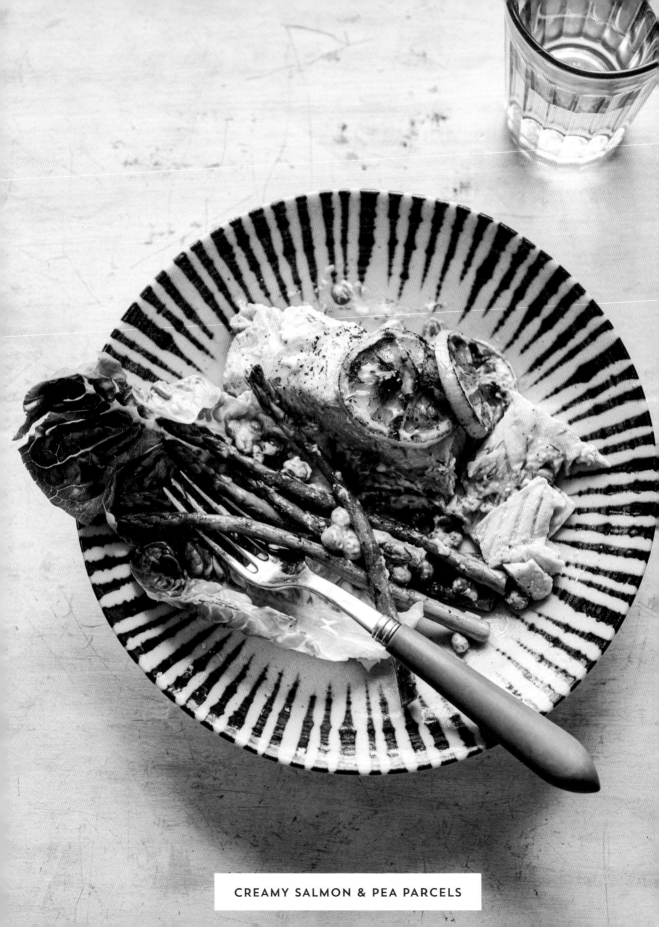

CREAMY SALMON & PEA PARCELS

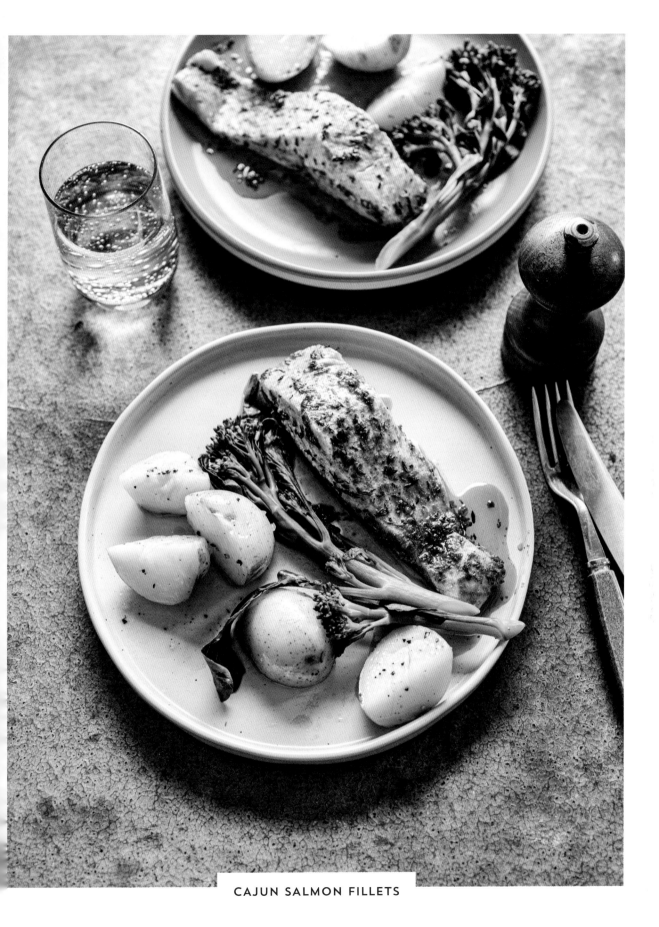

CAJUN SALMON FILLETS

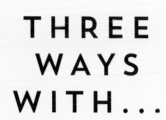

THREE WAYS WITH...

CAJUN SALMON FILLETS

Now that you've prepared your Cajun Salmon Fillets, what are you going to do with them? Here are three simple ideas for different ways of serving them that will keep mealtimes feeling fresh and different every time. Each meal serves 4.

CAJUN SALMON TACOS

1 x quantity Cajun Salmon Fillets
  (p.169)
8 taco shells
1 x 160g can sweetcorn, drained
1 tub shop-bought salsa
1 tub shop-bought guacamole (or
  use the recipe from my meal
  planner book)

1   Cook the salmon as per the instructions on page 169.
2   Once cooked, flake the salmon into a bowl and discard the skin.
3   Layer the tacos with the sweetcorn, salsa, guacamole and salmon. Serve while the salmon is still hot.

CAJUN SALMON SALAD

1 x quantity Cajun Salmon Fillets
  (p.169)
large bowl of mixed salad of
  your choice (I like salad leaves,
  sweetcorn, chopped boiled
  eggs, sliced cucumber, chopped
  tomatoes and sliced avocado)
1 x quantity Low-Fat Ranch
  Dressing (p.211)

1 Cook the salmon as per the instructions on page 169.
2 Dress the salad with the dressing and toss to
   combine, then divide the salad between 4 serving
   bowls and top each with a hot salmon fillet. Serve.

CAJUN SALMON WITH MANGE TOUT & NOODLES

1 x quantity Cajun Salmon Fillets
  (p.169)
2 nests wholewheat noodles
150g mange tout

1 Cook the salmon as per the instructions on page 169.
2 5 minutes before the salmon has finished cooking,
   add the noodles to a pan of boiling water over
   a medium heat and cook according to the pack
   instructions, until tender. Once cooked, drain
   through a colander.
3 Meanwhile, in a second pan of boiling water, cook
   the mange tout for 3–4 minutes, until tender. Once
   cooked, drain through a colander.
4 Divide the noodles and mange tout between 4
   serving plates and top each with a hot salmon fillet.
   Serve hot.

CREAMY TURKEY & MUSHROOM CARBONARA

PREP: 5 MINS **COOK:** 10 MINS **SERVES:** 4 **SUGAR:** 4.9G **KCAL:** 278

low-calorie cooking spray
1 cup (115g) frozen chopped onions
1 tsp frozen chopped garlic
6 turkey bacon rashers, finely chopped
2 cups (140g) white mushrooms, sliced
2 cups (400g) low-fat crème fraîche
½ cup (50g) pre-grated Parmesan cheese
salt and freshly ground pepper
300g wholewheat spaghetti, to serve

1 Spray a large saucepan with low-calorie cooking spray and place over a medium heat. Add the onions, garlic, chopped turkey bacon and sliced mushrooms and cook, stirring occasionally, for 6–8 minutes, until the vegetables are softened and the turkey bacon has cooked through.

> *If you are also making the Cajun Turkey and Pepper Meatloaf, cook the onions, garlic and peppers in a separate pan now.*

2 Add the crème fraîche and grated Parmesan and stir to combine. Cook for a further minute, then season to taste and remove from the heat.

Make it Veggie!
If you're making this for vegetarians, simply substitute the turkey rashers with vegetarian bacon rashers and cook in the same way.

TO SERVE

Cook the spaghetti according to packet instructions, until tender, then drain and add to the pan with the carbonara sauce, giving everything a good stir to ensure the pasta is coated in the sauce. Divide between serving bowls and serve hot.

TO FREEZE

Set the carbonara sauce aside to cool to room temperature, then transfer to a labelled freezer bag and freeze flat for up to 3 months.

TO COOK FROM FROZEN

Remove the carbonara sauce from the freezer and leave to defrost fully in the fridge, ideally overnight. Once defrosted tip the sauce into a large saucepan and place over a gentle heat, stirring occasionally, until piping hot all of the way through. While the sauce is heating, cook the spaghetti according to packet instructions and serve the dish as described in the *To Cook* section, left.

CAJUN TURKEY-AND-PEPPER MEATLOAF

PREP: 10 MINS **COOK:** 50 MINS–1 HR **SERVES:** 4 **SUGAR:** 9.9G **KCAL:** 293

low-calorie cooking spray
1 cup (115g) frozen chopped onions
2 tsp frozen chopped garlic
1 cup (175g) frozen mixed peppers
500g lean turkey mince
3 tsp Cajun seasoning
1 tbsp Worcestershire sauce
½ cup (25g) panko breadcrumbs
1 egg, beaten
1 tbsp tomato purée
2 tbsp reduced-salt-and-sugar
  tomato ketchup
1 tsp runny honey
1 tsp white wine vinegar
salt and freshly ground pepper

To serve
Lighter Serve: A big, leafy salad
Family Serve: Low-Cal Cheesy
Mash (p.202) and steamed
green veg

1 Spray a frying pan with low-calorie cooking spray and place over a medium heat. Add the onions, garlic and peppers and cook for 2–3 minutes, until the vegetables are soft. Remove the pan from the heat and set aside to cool.

> If you are also making the Creamy Turkey & Mushroom Carbonara, return to step 2 now while the vegetables are cooling.

2 Add the turkey mince, Cajun seasoning, Worcestershire sauce, breadcrumbs, egg, tomato purée and the cooked onion and pepper mixture to a large mixing bowl and season with a generous grinding of salt and pepper. Using your hands, mix all of the ingredients together until really well combined.

3 In a separate small bowl, combine the tomato ketchup, honey and white wine vinegar and set aside.

4 Line a baking tray with foil and tip the turkey mixture onto it. Using your hands, shape the mixture into a small loaf shape, roughly 15cm (6in) long x 7cm (2¾in) wide.

5 Using a pastry brush, brush the meatloaf all over with the ketchup and honey mixture.

TO COOK

Transfer the meatloaf to an oven preheated to 160°C/300°F/gas mark 3 and cook for 50 minutes–1 hour, until cooked through. Remove from the oven, cut into slices and serve hot, with your choice of accompaniments.

TO FREEZE

The meatloaf can either be frozen whole and uncooked by wrapping in a layer of clingfilm followed by a layer of foil and freeze flat for up to 3 months, or cooked first as per the *To Cook* instructions, left, then left to cool and frozen in individual slices.

TO COOK FROM FROZEN

Depending on how you froze the meatloaf (see *To Freeze*, left), remove the whole meatloaf or as many individual slices as you need from the freezer and leave to defrost in the fridge, ideally overnight. If the meatloaf is whole and uncooked, cook as per the *To Cook* instructions, left. If you are reheating individual slices, simply reheat on high in the microwave for 2–3 minutes, until piping hot all of the way through.

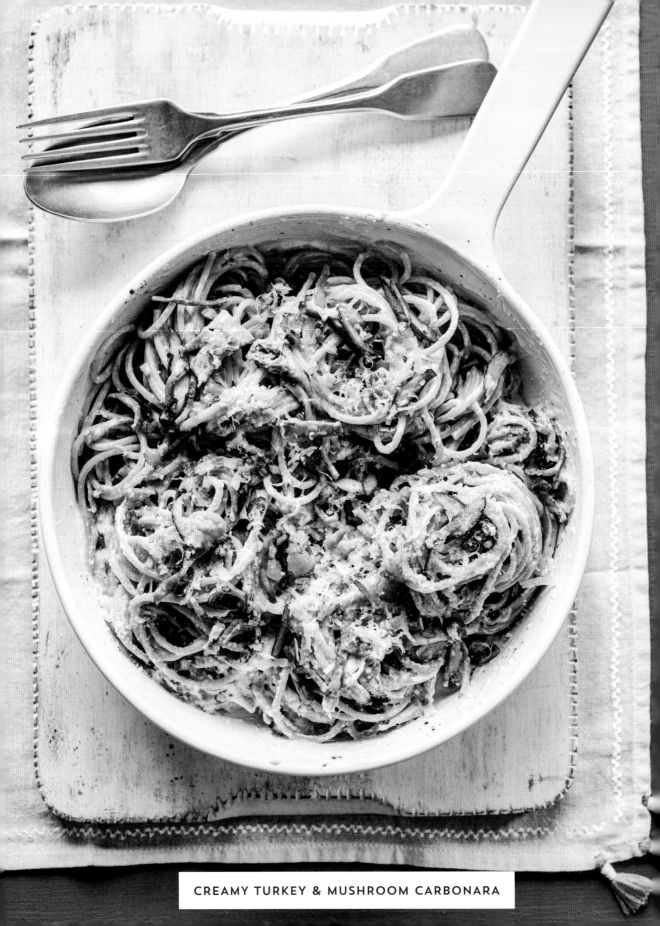

CREAMY TURKEY & MUSHROOM CARBONARA

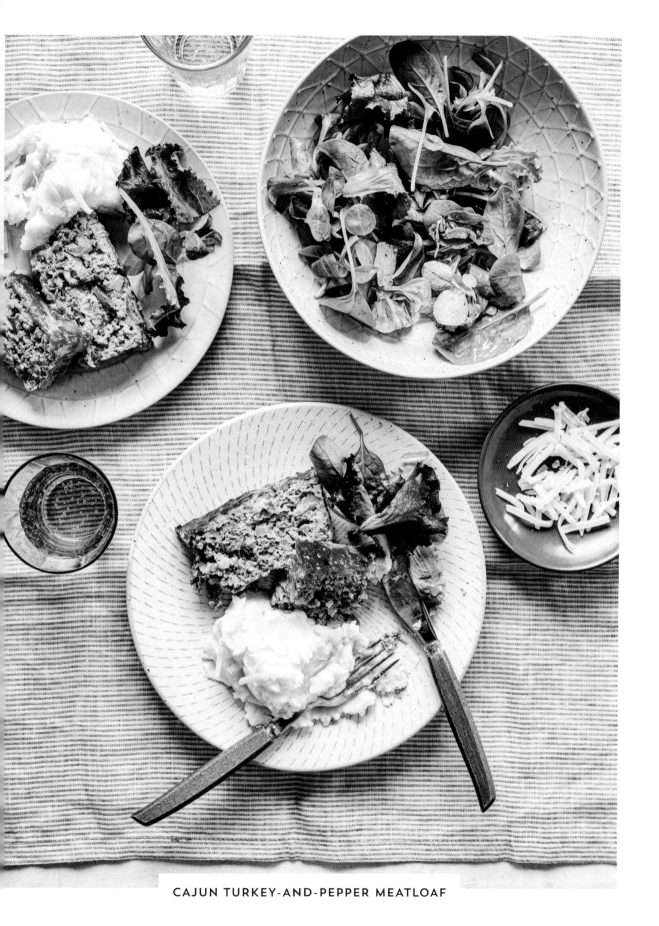

CAJUN TURKEY-AND-PEPPER MEATLOAF

TURKEY TAGINE

PREP: 10 MINS **COOK:** 35 MINS **SERVES:** 4 **SUGAR:** 20G **KCAL:** 312

1 tbsp olive oil

3 turkey breast steaks, cut into bite-sized pieces

1 cup (115g) frozen chopped onions

1 tsp frozen chopped garlic

1 tsp frozen chopped ginger

2 tbsp tagine seasoning (available in supermarkets)

1 tbsp tomato purée

2 x 400g cans chopped tomatoes

1 cup (240ml) low-sodium chicken stock

1 x 400g can chickpeas, drained

10 dried apricots, finely chopped (optional)

salt and freshly ground pepper

To serve

Lighter Serve: Cauliflower rice (p.203) and a scattering of chopped fresh coriander

Family Serve: Couscous and Light-And-Easy Paprika Flatbreads (p.209) alongside

1. Heat the oil in a large saucepan over a medium heat. Add the turkey and cook, stirring, for around 5 minutes, until browned. Using a slotted spoon, transfer the turkey from the pan to a bowl and set aside. Keep the pan on the heat.

2. Add the onions, garlic and ginger and cook, stirring, for 2–3 minutes, until the onions are softened.

3. Add the tagine seasoning, tomato purée, chopped tomatoes and chicken stock to the pan and stir to combine. Bring the mixture to the boil, then reduce the heat to a gentle simmer and leave to thicken and reduce for 15 minutes, stirring occasionally.

> If you are also making the Lamb Chops with Salsa Verde, chop the herbs and assemble the salsa verde now, while the tagine is bubbling away.

4. After 15 minutes, return the turkey to the pan and add the chickpeas, apricots, if using, and a grinding of salt and pepper, then leave to cook for another 10 minutes, stirring occasionally, to allow the flavours to develop. Remove the pan from the heat.

Make it Veggie!

Substitute the chicken breast for plant-based chicken-style pieces. If you are doing this, skip step 1 of the recipe and add the plant-based chicken with the chickpeas in step 4.

TO SERVE

The tagine is now ready to serve with your choice of accompaniments.

TO FREEZE

Leave the tagine to cool to room temperature, then transfer to a large, labelled freezer bag and freeze flat for up to 3 months.

TO REHEAT FROM FROZEN

This can be fully defrosted and then reheated in a pan or cooked from frozen. If cooking from frozen, tip into a pan, cover with a lid and place over a low heat. Cook, removing the lid occasionally and breaking up with a wooden spoon as the mixture defrosts, until fully defrosted and piping hot all of the way through.

LAMB CHOPS WITH SALSA VERDE

PREP: 10 MINS **COOK:** 6 MINS **SERVES:** 4 **SUGAR:** 0.5G **KCAL:** 398

The salsa verde in this dish packs real flavour, so is more than worth the effort of chopping all of the fresh herbs. When making it, I like to double-up, so that I can use up all of the herbs and not have to worry about waste. This is a wonderful dinner party dish and, if the sauce is made ahead, the meat can be cooked and on the table in less than 10 minutes, taking all of the stress out of entertaining and giving you more time to enjoy with your guests.

8 lamb chops

For the salsa verde:

1 large handful fresh parsley, roughly chopped

1 large handful fresh coriander, roughly chopped

1 large handful fresh mint, roughly chopped

2 tbsp small capers, drained, rinsed and roughly chopped

1 tsp garlic purée

1 tsp Dijon mustard

2 tsp red wine vinegar

6 tbsp olive oil

salt and freshly ground pepper

To serve

Lighter Serve: Boiled new potatoes and steamed asparagus

Family Serve: Buttered new potatoes and pan-fried asparagus

1 Put all the ingredients for the salsa verde except the olive oil in a large mixing bowl. Add the olive oil, a tablespoon at a time, stirring between each addition to allow the mixture to emulsify. Season with salt and freshly ground pepper to taste.

TO COOK

Preheat the grill to high and line a grill pan with foil. Lay the lamb chops on the grill pan and season on both sides with salt and pepper. Place under the hot grill for 3 minutes, then turn the chops and cook on the other side for another 3 minutes. Serve the chops with the salsa verde alongside for spooning over.

TO FREEZE

Transfer the uncooked lamb chops to a large, labelled freezer bag, but do not seal. Transfer the salsa verde to a smaller freezer bag and seal, then place this bag into the larger bag with the lamb. Seal the larger bag and freeze flat for up to 3 months.

TO COOK FROM FROZEN

Remove the bag containing the lamb chops and salsa verde from the freezer and leave to fully defrost in the fridge, ideally overnight. Dab the defrosted lamb chops with kitchen paper, then cook under the grill as described in the *To Cook* section, left. Serve the chops with the salsa verde alongside for spooning over.

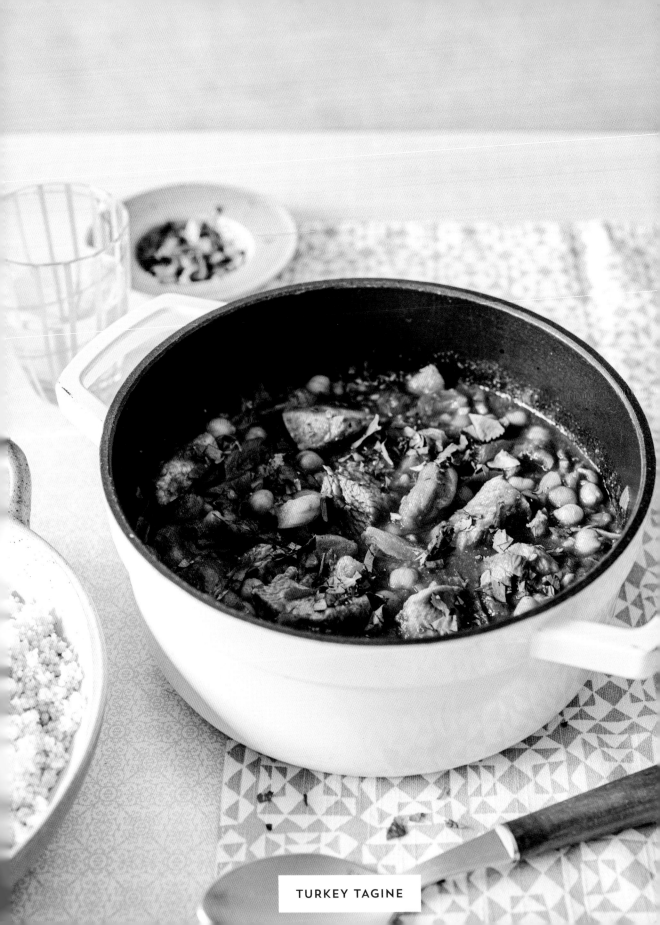

TURKEY TAGINE

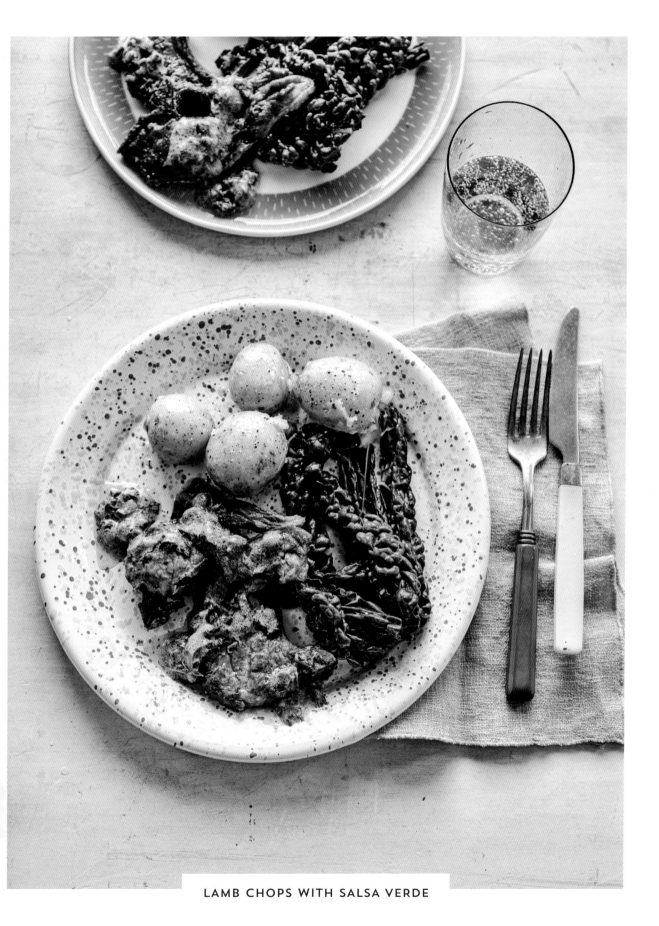

LAMB CHOPS WITH SALSA VERDE

BEETROOT & FETA ORZOTTO

PREP: 5-10 MINS **COOK:** 15 MINS **SERVES:** 4 **SUGAR:** 7.2G **KCAL:** 463

This wonderfully pink-hued dish is packed full of the vibrant earthy flavours of beetroot and is as much of a feast for the eyes as it is for the tastebuds. Orzo, meaning barley in Italian, gets its name from its small grain shape, but is actually a form of pasta.

low-calorie cooking spray
1 cup (115g) frozen chopped onions
2 tsp frozen chopped garlic
1 x 250g pack cooked beetroot, roughly chopped
2 cups (400g) orzo
3 cups (720ml) low-sodium vegetable stock

On day of serving:
juice of 1 lemon
100g low-fat feta cheese, crumbled

1 Spray a large saucepan with low-calorie cooking spray and place over a medium heat. Add the onions and garlic and cook, stirring continuously, for 2–3 minutes until soft.
2 Meanwhile, put the beetroot into a food processor or freestanding blender and pulse briefly to break it down. You still want some texture to the beetroot, so do not blend until smooth.
3 When the onions and garlic are soft, add the orzo to the pan and stir to combine, then add the vegetable stock and beetroot to the pan and stir again. Bring the mixture to the boil, then reduce the heat to a simmer and leave to cook, stirring occasionally, for 8 minutes

---

TO COOK

Continue cooking the orzotto mixture for another 4 minutes, until the orzo is tender. Remove from the heat and stir through the lemon juice and half of the feta. Portion into bowls and serve hot, garnished with the remaining feta.

TO FREEZE

Remove the orzotto mixture from the heat and leave to cool to room temperature, then transfer to a large, labelled freezer bag and freeze flat for up to 3 months.

TO REHEAT FROM FROZEN

This can be defrosted in the fridge overnight and then reheated in a pan until piping hot, or cooked from frozen. If cooking from frozen, tip the frozen orzotto into a large saucepan, cover with a lid and place over a low heat. Cook the mixture, removing the lid occasionally and breaking it up with a wooden spoon as the mixture defrosts, until it is fully defrosted and piping hot all of the way through. Remove from the heat and stir through the lemon juice and half of the feta. Portion into bowls and serve hot, garnished with the remaining feta.

OVEN-BAKED SUNDRIED TOMATO RISOTTO

PREP: 10 MINS **COOK:** 25 MINS **SERVES:** 4 **SUGAR:** 11G **KCAL:** 488

While standing over a pot of rice and stirring until cooked to perfection can feel like a real achievement, there are times when you want the comfort of a risotto without the effort. This oven-baked version is lighter and lower calorie than a traditional risotto, without sacrificing on any of the wonderful creamy texture.

low-calorie cooking spray
1 cup (115g) frozen chopped onions
1 tsp frozen chopped garlic
2 cups (300g) Arborio rice
2 tbsp sundried tomato pesto
1 x 500g carton passata
3½ cups (840ml) low-sodium vegetable stock
1 tbsp low-fat mascarpone cheese
salt and freshly ground pepper
pre-grated Parmesan cheese, to serve

1 Preheat the oven to 200°C/400°F/gas mark 6.
2 Spray a large, ovenproof saucepan with a lid with low-calorie cooking spray and place over a medium heat. Add the onions and garlic and cook, stirring continuously, for 2–3 minutes, until soft.
3 Add the rice to the pan and cook, stirring continuously, for 2–3 minutes to toast the grains and coat them in the cooking spray.
4 Add the pesto, passata and vegetable stock and stir to combine. Bring the mixture just to the boil, then cover with a lid and transfer the pan to the oven for 10–15 minutes, until the rice is almost tender.

TO COOK

Continue to cook the risotto in the oven for another 5 minutes, until the rice is tender, then remove from the oven and stir through the mascarpone. Season the risotto to taste and portion into serving bowls. Serve hot, garnished with grated Parmesan.

TO FREEZE

Remove the risotto from the oven now, just before the rice is tender and stir through the mascarpone. Set aside to cool to room temperature, then transfer the risotto to a large, labelled freezer bag and freeze flat for up to 3 months.

TO REHEAT FROM FROZEN

Remove the risotto from the freezer and leave to defrost fully in the fridge, ideally overnight. Once defrosted, transfer the risotto to a large saucepan and heat over a low heat, stirring continuously, until piping hot all of the way through. If the mixture is too thick, add a little water to loosen. Serve hot, garnished with grated Parmesan.

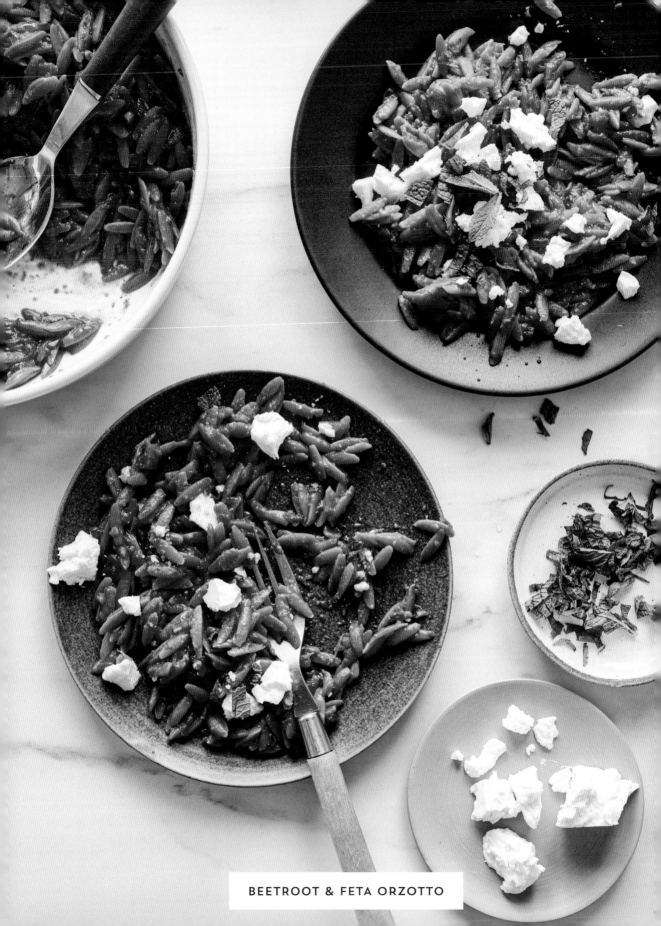

BEETROOT & FETA ORZOTTO

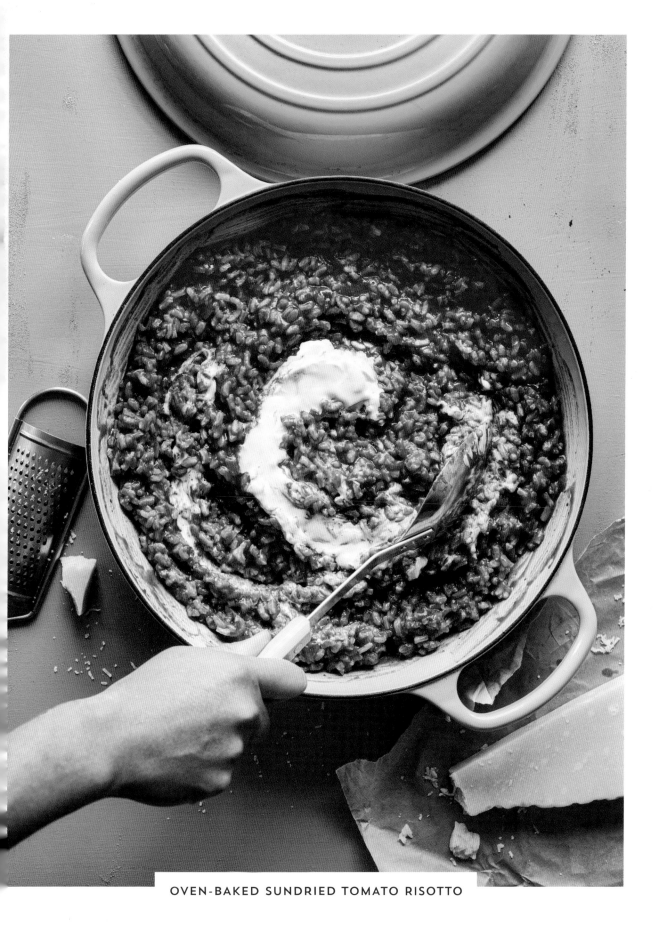

OVEN-BAKED SUNDRIED TOMATO RISOTTO

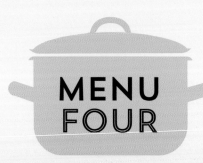

MENU FOUR

3 FOR THE FRIDGE,
3 FOR THE FREEZER

Are you ready to batch three family meals for the week ahead and three to store in the freezer for another time in just 45 minutes? You will be making three recipes, each of which is doubled-up to feed eight people, so you simply need to split the recipe into two family meals before freezing one and putting the other in the fridge for the week ahead. The recipes are a mixture of cooked and no-cook freezer-bag meals, so while one recipe is bubbling away on the stove or cooking in the oven, you can be making the next meal ready for the fridge and freezer.

The shopping list on the opposite page includes everything you need and I have scaled up the ingredients for you so you don't need to worry about doubling the recipe. Simply buy what's on the shopping list and you will have everything you need to make the six meals. Once you have your shopping, lay the ingredients out into piles according to the groupings overleaf, so you have exactly what you need for each recipe to hand. Then simply follow the numbered guide and you can't go wrong!

Don't panic if this takes you more than 45 minutes the first time you cook it – you will get quicker each time you make it. So, roll up your sleeves, get cooking and think about the time you will be saving yourself in the future!

YOU WILL BE MAKING:

ROSEMARY & GARLIC ROAST POTATOES

HONEY & MUSTARD SAUSAGE TRAYBAKE

HARISSA MARINATED CHICKEN

SHOPPING LIST

Fresh

1 x 1.5kg bag Maris Piper potatoes

1 x 1kg bag new potatoes

4 red onions

1 x 250g pack cherry tomatoes

16 low-fat pork sausages

1 x 500g pot low-fat natural yoghurt

2 lemons

8 skinless, boneless chicken breasts

Frozen

1 x 75g pack frozen chopped garlic

Storecupboard

1 x 500g bag plain flour

olive oil

1 x 180g jar wholegrain mustard

1 x 340g bottle runny honey

1 x 90g jar harissa paste

1 jar dried rosemary

salt and pepper

INGREDIENTS

GET ORGANISED! Before you start cooking, make sure that your kitchen surfaces are cleared down, then lay all the ingredients out in individual piles according to the groupings below.

ROSEMARY & GARLIC ROAST POTATOES

1.4kg Maris Piper potatoes
2 tbsp plain flour
4 tsp dried rosemary
4 tbsp olive oil
4 tsp frozen chopped garlic
salt and freshly ground pepper

HONEY & MUSTARD SAUSAGE TRAYBAKE

800g new potatoes, halved if large
4 tbsp wholegrain mustard
4 tbsp runny honey
4 tbsp olive oil
4 red onions, roughly chopped
20 cherry tomatoes
16 low-fat pork sausages
salt and freshly ground pepper

HARISSA MARINATED CHICKEN

2 cups (440g) low-fat natural yoghurt
4 tsp harissa paste
2 tsp frozen chopped garlic
juice of 2 lemons
8 skinless, boneless chicken breasts, cut into strips
salt and freshly ground pepper

METHOD

ROSEMARY & GARLIC ROAST POTATOES

1 Peel the potatoes and cut into halves or quarters, depending on their size.
2 Put the potatoes in a large saucepan with a lid and pour over cold water to cover. Place the pan over a medium heat, cover with a lid and bring to the boil. Once boiling, reduce the heat to a gentle simmer and leave to cook for 5 minutes while you get started with the Honey & Mustard Sausage Traybake.

HONEY & MUSTARD SAUSAGE TRAYBAKE

3 Put the new potatoes in a large saucepan with a lid and pour over cold water to cover. Place the pan over a medium heat, cover with a lid and bring to the boil. Once boiling, reduce the heat to a gentle simmer and leave to cook for 5 minutes.
4 While the potatoes are cooking, combine the mustard, honey, olive oil and a grinding of salt and pepper in a small bowl and set aside.
5 Set 2 large, labelled freezer bags side-by-side on the counter. Into each bag add half of the chopped red onions and cherry tomatoes and 8 of the sausages.
6 Pour half of the mustard sauce into each bag and gently massage to ensure the sausages and vegetables are coated in the sauce. Set aside.

ROSEMARY & GARLIC ROAST POTATOES CONTINUED...

7 Drain the potatoes through a colander and leave to steam-dry for a couple of minutes.
8 Return the potatoes to the pan, off the heat, and sprinkle over the flour. Add the rosemary, olive oil, garlic and a generous grinding of salt and pepper and toss the pan to coat the potatoes in the flour, herbs, oil and garlic.
9 Line a baking tray with foil and turn the potatoes out onto it. Set aside to cool.

HONEY & MUSTARD SAUSAGE TRAYBAKE CONTINUED...

10 Drain the potatoes through a colander and set aside to cool.

CONTINUED OVERLEAF...

HARISSA MARINATED CHICKEN

11 Add the yoghurt, harissa, garlic and lemon juice to a large mixing bowl and stir to combine.

12 Add the chicken strips to the bowl and stir to coat well with the yoghurt and harissa mixture.

13 Transfer half of the chicken mixture to a large, labelled freezer bag and freeze flat for up to 3 months. Put the other half in a container with a lid and transfer to the fridge to use in the week ahead.

HONEY & MUSTARD SAUSAGE TRAYBAKE CONTINUED...

14 Divide the cooled new potatoes equally between the two freezer bags containing the vegetable and sausage mixture. Seal the bags and place one in the freezer, flat, for up to 3 months, and the other in the fridge to use in the week ahead.

ROSEMARY & GARLIC ROAST POTATOES CONTINUED...

15 Put half of the cooled, part-cooked roast potatoes in a container with a lid and transfer to the fridge to use in the week ahead. Leave the remaining roast potatoes on the baking tray and transfer to the freezer to part-freeze for 2 hours. Remove from the freezer and transfer to a large, labelled freezer bag. Freeze flat for up to 3 months.

Congratulations!
You have just made six meals!
Three for the week ahead
and three for the freezer.

WHEN YOU COME TO COOK

Once cooked, all of these meals are best fully defrosted before cooking. All reheated meals should reach a temperature of 74°C/165°F. Always make sure any reheated food is piping hot before serving. Cooking instructions for each dish are given below.

ROSEMARY & GARLIC ROAST POTATOES

FROM THE FRIDGE

Preheat the oven to 180°C/350°F/gas mark 4. Spread the potatoes out on a foil-lined baking tray and transfer to the oven to cook for 35 minutes, until golden and crunchy.

FROM THE FREEZER

These can be cooked straight from frozen. Preheat the oven to 180°C/350°F/gas mark 4. Spread the potatoes out on a foil-lined baking tray and transfer to the oven to cook for 50 minutes, until golden and crunchy.

HONEY & MUSTARD SAUSAGE TRAYBAKE

FROM THE FRIDGE

Preheat the oven to 180°C/350°F/gas mark 4. Tip the sausage and vegetable mixture into a roasting tin in an even layer, then transfer to the oven to cook for around 30 minutes, until the sausages are cooked through and the vegetables are tender.

FROM THE FREEZER

Remove the sausage and vegetable bag from the freezer and leave to fully defrost in the fridge, ideally overnight. Once defrosted, cook as directed in the *From the Fridge* section, above.

HARISSA MARINATED CHICKEN

FROM THE FRIDGE

Preheat the oven to 180°C/350°F/gas mark 4 and line a baking tray with foil. Shake any excess marinade from the chicken and lay the strips on the baking tray, then transfer to the oven to cook for 20 minutes, until tender and cooked through.

FROM THE FREEZER

Remove the chicken from the freezer and leave to fully defrost in the fridge, ideally overnight. Once defrosted, cook as directed in the *From the Fridge* section, above.

To serve

Lighter Serve: Salad, wholemeal pitta breads and hummus
Family Serve: Salad, hummus, low-fat feta cheese and wholemeal pitta breads

SIDES & SAUCES

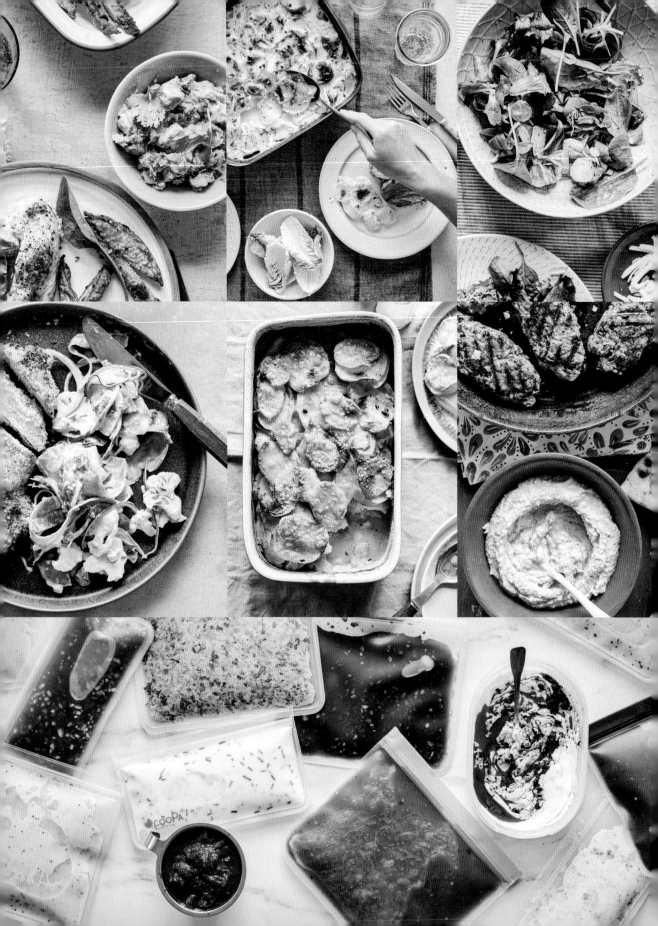

SIDES & SAUCES

Use the recipes in this chapter to dress up your meals and make them feel complete. In the previous chapters, you will have seen that most of my recipes have lighter and family serving suggestions and many of the recipes for these are from this chapter.

Potatoes have got a bad reputation when it comes to eating lean, but my recipes for Lighter Dauphinoise Potatoes (p.198), Boulangère Potatoes (p.199) and Low-Cal Cheesy Mash (p.202) mean that you can still enjoy your favourite dishes, even if you are trying to watch what you eat. I couldn't have a sides chapter without chips, so there are also a couple of recipes for lighter, oven-baked versions, too.

To complete the recipes in the Fakeaway chapter (p.82–113) you will find lighter versions of takeaway classics, such as Bombay Potatoes (p.196) Light-And-Easy Naan Breads (p.208) and Cauliflower Rice (p.203), so that you can make curry night a real feast without worrying about the calories.

The sauces and dressings in this chapter can be added to simple salads and grilled fish or meats to make them feel really special. I keep a pot of the Low-Fat Blue Cheese Dressing (p.210) in my fridge at all times to use as a dip, which encourages me to eat more healthy veg every day.

BOMBAY POTATOES

PREP: 10 MINS **COOK:** 45–55 MINS **SERVES:** 4 **SUGAR:** 4.3G **KCAL:** 237

These punchy potatoes make a great alternative to rice when served with a curry. They can go straight from the freezer to the oven, so are a brilliant, low-fuss option for Friday night curries that the whole family will enjoy.

600g white potatoes (Maris Piper work well), peeled and chopped into halves or quarters, depending on the size
1 red onion, roughly chopped
2 tbsp tikka masala spice paste
2 tbsp olive oil
salt and freshly ground pepper

1   Put the potatoes in a large saucepan and cover with cold water. Place the pan over a high heat and cover with a lid. Bring to the boil, then remove the lid and reduce the heat to a simmer. Cook for 5 minutes, then drain the potatoes through a colander.

If you are also making the Paprika Hasselback Potatoes, parboil those in a separate pan at the same time.

2   Return the pan to the heat and tip the drained potatoes back in. Cook the potatoes, stirring continuously to prevent them from sticking, for 1 minute, until dry. Remove the pan from the heat.

3   Add the red onion, tikka masala spice paste, olive oil and a generous grinding of salt and pepper to the pan and stir to combine with the potatoes. Tip the potatoes into a large roasting tin and spread out in an even layer.

TO COOK

Transfer the roasting tin to an oven preheated to 180°C/350°F/gas mark 4 and cook for 40–50 minutes, turning halfway through cooking, until crisp and golden. Serve hot.

TO FREEZE

Set the roasting tin aside until the potatoes have cooled to room temperature, then transfer the tin to the freezer for 1 hour to allow the potatoes to part-freeze. After an hour, transfer the potatoes to a large, labelled freezer bag and freeze flat for up to 3 months.

TO COOK FROM FROZEN

These can be cooked directly from frozen. Tip the frozen potatoes into a roasting tin and cook in an oven preheated to 180°C/350°F/gas mark 4 for 45–55 minutes, until crisp, golden and piping hot all of the way through. Serve hot.

PAPRIKA HASSELBACK POTATOES

PREP: 10 MINS **COOK:** 50 MINS **SERVES:** 4 **SUGAR:** 2G **KCAL:** 217

Slicing the fan pattern into these potatoes may seem like a faff, but the wonderfully crisp end result is more than worth the effort. Once prepped and in the freezer, these can be cooked straight from frozen, so are great for days when you're too busy to make anything from scratch. I like to serve these with a dollop of low-fat sour cream and a sprinkling of chives for a real treat of a side dish.

16 medium new potatoes
1–2 tsp paprika
2–3 tbsp olive oil
2 tsp frozen chopped garlic, on
  day of cooking
salt and freshly ground pepper

1   Place a potato in the hollowed-out 'bowl' of a wooden spoon and use a sharp knife to carefully make cuts along their width at roughly 3mm (⅛in) intervals. The spoon should prevent you from cutting all of the way through the potato. Repeat until all of the potatoes are sliced.

2   Put the prepared potatoes into a large saucepan and cover with cold water. Place the pan over a high heat and cover with a lid. Bring to the boil, then remove the lid and reduce the heat to a simmer. Cook for 5 minutes, then drain the potatoes through a colander.

3   Return the potatoes to the pan, off the heat, and add the paprika, olive oil and a generous grinding of salt and pepper. Toss the potatoes in the pan to ensure they are well coated in the oil and spices.

TO COOK

Tip the spiced potatoes onto a foil-lined baking tray and spread out in an even layer. Transfer to an oven preheated to 180°C/350°F/gas mark 4 and cook for 30 minutes. Add the garlic to the baking tray and toss with the potatoes to coat, then return to the oven for another 10 minutes until crisp and golden.

TO FREEZE

Set the spiced, par-boiled potatoes aside to cool to room temperature, then transfer to a large, labelled freezer bag and freeze flat for up to 3 months.

TO COOK FROM FROZEN

These can be cooked directly from frozen. Tip the frozen, spiced potatoes onto a foil-lined baking tray and spread out in an even layer. Transfer to an oven preheated to 180°C/350°F/gas mark 4 and cook for 40 minutes. Add the garlic to the baking tray and toss with the potatoes to coat, then return to the oven for another 10 minutes until crisp, golden and piping hot.

LIGHTER DAUPHINOISE POTATOES

PREP: 15 MINS **COOK:** 1 HR **SERVES:** 4 **SUGAR:** 4.1G **KCAL:** 249

Dauphinoise potatoes are always a treat, so I wanted to find a way of enjoying them without worrying about all the extra calories – this is the result! You'll be amazed by how rich and creamy these are, despite being far lighter than a traditional dauphinoise.

750g Maris Piper potatoes
1 cup (200g) low-fat crème fraîche
1 cup (120ml) semi-skimmed milk
¼ cup (60ml) low-sodium vegetable stock
1 tsp dried thyme
2 tsp frozen chopped garlic
salt and freshly ground pepper

1 Preheat the oven to 180°C/350°F/gas mark 4. Peel the potatoes and slice as thinly as possible, if possible using a mandolin or the slicing blade of a food processor.

> If you are also making the Boulangère Potatoes, slice the potatoes for both dishes at the same time.

2 Put the crème fraîche, milk, vegetable stock, dried thyme and frozen garlic in a large pan with a generous grinding of salt and pepper and place over a low heat, stirring occasionally, until the mixture is warmed but not boiling.
3 While the crème fraîche and stock mixture is warming, arrange the sliced potatoes in a shallow baking dish in even layers.
4 Once warmed, pour the crème fraîche and stock mixture over the potatoes.

TO COOK

Carefully transfer the dish to the oven to cook for 1 hour, until the potatoes are tender and the top layer is golden. Serve hot.

TO FREEZE

Carefully transfer the dish to the oven to cook for 20 minutes, then remove from the oven and leave to cool to room temperature. Once cooled, cover the dish with a layer of clingfilm followed by a layer of foil, label and freeze for up to 3 months.

TO COOK FROM FROZEN

Remove from the freezer and leave to defrost fully in the fridge, ideally overnight. Once defrosted, remove the clingfilm but re-cover the dish with the foil, then transfer to an oven preheated to 180°C/350°F/gas mark 4 for 30 minutes. Remove the foil and return the potatoes to the oven for a final 10 minutes, until the potatoes are tender and the top layer is golden.

BOULANGÈRE POTATOES

PREP: 10 MINS **COOK:** 1 HR **SERVES:** 6 **SUGAR:** 1G **KCAL:** 224

This dish is similar to a dauphinoise, but uses stock instead of cream which means the dish is both lighter and kinder on the waistline.

750g Maris Piper potatoes
low-calorie cooking spray
1 cup (115g) frozen chopped
  onions
1 tsp dried thyme
1¼ cups (300ml) low-sodium
  vegetable stock
1 cup (70g) pre-grated Parmesan
  cheese

1 Preheat the oven to 180°C/350°F/gas mark 4. Peel the potatoes and slice as thinly as possible, if possible using a mandolin or the slicing blade of a food processor.
2 Spray a large saucepan with low-calorie cooking spray and place over a medium heat. Add the onions and thyme and cook, stirring continuously, for 2–3 minutes, until soft.
3 Arrange half of the sliced potatoes in a shallow baking dish in an even layer, then spoon the onion and thyme mixture over the top of the potatoes.
4 Top with the remaining potatoes in an even layer, then pour over the vegetable stock.
5 Scatter the grated Parmesan over the top of the dish.

TO COOK

Carefully transfer the dish to the oven to cook for 1 hour, until the potatoes are tender and the top layer is golden. Serve hot.

TO FREEZE

Carefully transfer the dish to the oven to cook for 20 minutes, then remove from the oven and leave to cool to room temperature. Once cooled, cover the dish with a layer of clingfilm followed by a layer of foil, label and freeze for up to 3 months.

TO COOK FROM FROZEN

Remove from the freezer and leave to defrost fully in the fridge, ideally overnight. Once defrosted, remove the foil and clingfilm, then transfer the dish to an oven preheated to 180°C/350°F/gas mark 4 for 40 minutes, until the potatoes are tender and the top layer is golden.

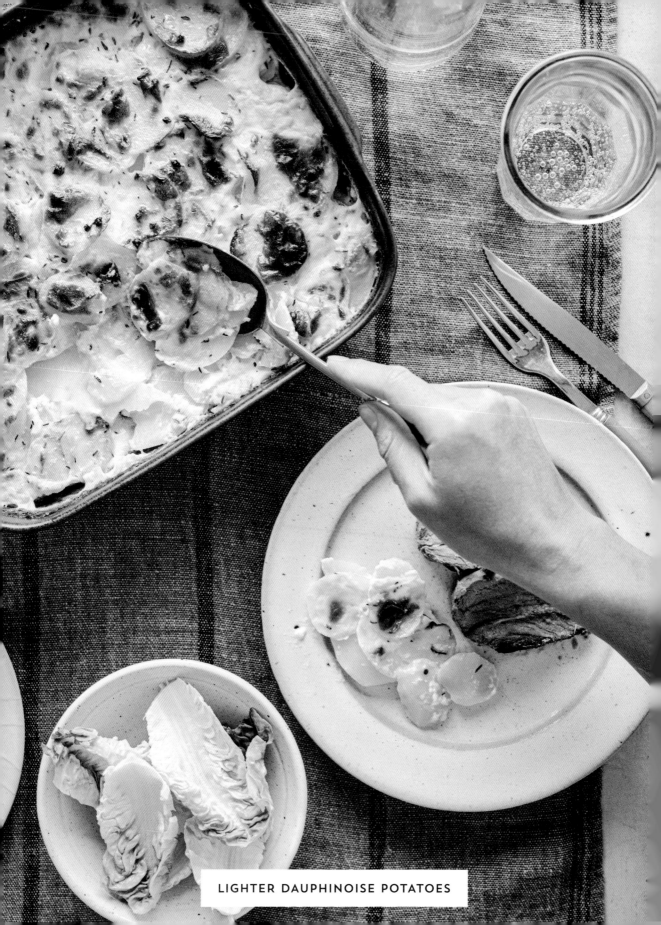

LIGHTER DAUPHINOISE POTATOES

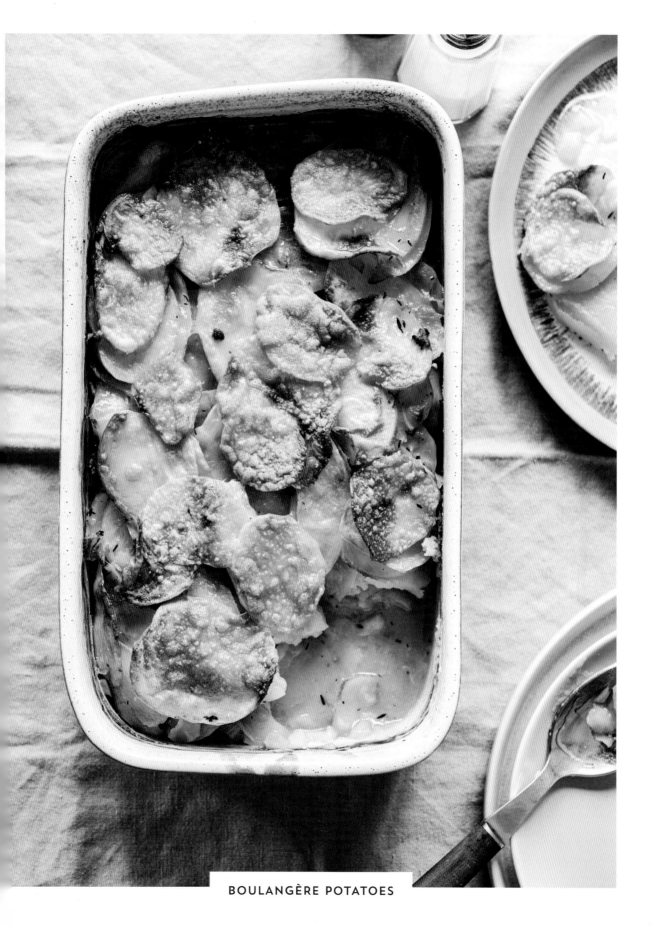

BOULANGÈRE POTATOES

LOW-CAL CHEESY MASH

PREP: 5 MINS **COOK:** 20 MINS **SERVES:** 4 **SUGAR:** 3.9G **KCAL:** 190

No matter how healthy you are trying to be, there are times when we all need a little comfort food – and in my house, that means mash! The following recipe offers all the hug-in-a-bowl comfort you could want, but is just that little bit lighter. If you're not a cheese fan, simply omit it from the recipe.

500g white potatoes, peeled and cut into small chunks
¾ cup (165g) low-fat natural yoghurt
¾ cup (80g) low-fat, pre-grated cheddar cheese
½ cup (120ml) low-sodium vegetable stock
salt and freshly ground pepper

1 Put the potatoes in a large saucepan with a lid and pour over cold water to cover. Place over a high heat, cover with a lid and bring to the boil, then remove the lid and reduce the heat to a simmer. Leave to cook for around 15 minutes, until tender. Then drain through a colander and leave to steam-dry for a couple of minutes.

> If you are also making the Cauliflower Rice, prepare it now while the potatoes are cooking.

2 Return the potatoes to the pan, off the heat, and mash until as smooth as possible. Add the yoghurt and grated cheese and stir to combine, then add the stock and stir again until smooth. Season to taste.

TO SERVE

The cheesy mash is now ready to serve.

TO FREEZE

Set aside to cool to room temperature, then transfer the mash to a large, labelled freezer bag (or several smaller bags if you would like to freeze in smaller portions) and freeze flat for up to 3 months.

TO REHEAT FROM FROZEN

Remove the mash from the freezer and leave to defrost fully in the fridge, ideally overnight. The mash can be reheated in the microwave by cooking on high for 4 minutes, or transferred to a baking dish and reheated in an oven preheated to 180°C/350°F/gas mark 4 for 15–20 minutes, until piping hot all of the way through.

CAULIFLOWER RICE

PREP: 5 MINS **COOK:** 5 MINS **SERVES:** 4 **SUGAR:** 3.6G **KCAL:** 51

This is a great low-calorie alternative to rice for anyone who wants to keep their side dishes carb-free. It makes a wonderful accompaniment to any of the curry dishes in this book.

1 large or 2 small cauliflowers,
    leaves trimmed
salt and freshly ground pepper

1 Cut the cauliflower into florets, removing and discarding the tough stalk as you do so.
2 Put the cauliflower florets in a food processor and pulse to a rice texture. Be careful not to pulse too finely as you still want the cauliflower to have some bite. Season with salt and pepper.

TO COOK

Transfer the cauliflower rice to a microwavable bowl and add a couple of tablespoons of water. Cover with clingfilm and microwave on high for 2 minutes, then stir the rice and cook for 1 minute more. The cauliflower rice is now ready to serve.

TO FREEZE

Transfer the uncooked rice to a large, labelled freezer bag (or several smaller bags if you would like to freeze in smaller portions) and freeze flat for up to 3 months.

TO COOK FROM FROZEN

Remove the cauliflower rice from the freezer and crumble into a microwaveable bowl. Cover with clingfilm and microwave on high for 2 minutes, then stir the rice and cook for 1 minute more. The cauliflower rice is now ready to serve.

SKIN-ON CHIPS

PREP: 8 MINS **COOK:** 35 MINS **SERVES:** 4 **SUGAR:** 4.5G **KCAL:** 576

Making chips at home and baking them in the oven is far healthier than buying them ready-cooked or using the deep-fat fryer. I like to keep the skins on for extra fibre. When cutting your chips, think chunky chip-shop sized chips as oppose to fries and you can't go wrong.

6 large white potatoes
1 tbsp plain flour
4 tbsp vegetable oil

1. Wash the potatoes, then cut into chunky chips with a sharp knife.
2. Put the chips in a large pan and pour over cold water to cover. Place over a high heat, cover with a lid and bring to the boil, then remove the lid and reduce the heat to a simmer. Cook for 3 minutes, then drain through a colander and leave to steam-dry for a couple of minutes.
3. Return the chips to the pan, off the heat, then add the flour and oil and toss to combine.
4. Tip the chips onto a foil-lined baking tray and spread out in an even layer. It is important that the chips are not on top of each other as they will not crisp in the oven if they are.

TO COOK

Transfer the chips to an oven preheated to 200°C/400°F/gas mark 6 for 30 minutes, until crisp and golden. Serve hot.

TO FREEZE

Set the par-boiled chips aside to cool to room temperature. Once cooled, cover the baking tray and transfer to the freezer for 2 hours to allow the chips to firm up. Transfer the part-frozen chips to a large, labelled freezer bag and freeze flat for up to 3 months.

TO COOK FROM FROZEN

The chips can be cooked directly from frozen. Tip the chips onto a foil-lined baking tray and spread out in an even layer, then transfer to an oven preheated to 200°C/400°F/gas mark 6 for 40 minutes, until crisp, golden and piping hot all of the way through.

PIRI-PIRI SWEET POTATO CHIPS

PREP: 5 MINS **COOK:** 35 MINS **SERVES:** 4 **SUGAR:** 26G **KCAL:** 280

Sweet potatoes are higher in nutrients than white potatoes and, as their name suggests, are naturally sweet meaning that children love them. If members of your family aren't fans of spice, then leave out the piri-piri seasoning or substitute it with dried thyme or rosemary instead.

2 large sweet potatoes (approx. 730g), peeled and cut into chunky chips
1 tbsp plain flour
2 tbsp piri-piri seasoning
2 tsp frozen chopped garlic
3 tbsp olive oil

1 Put the sweet potato chips in a large pan and pour over cold water to cover. Place over a high heat, cover with a lid and bring to the boil, then remove the lid and reduce the heat to a simmer. Cook for 3 minutes, then drain through a colander and leave to steam-dry for a couple of minutes.

2 Return the chips to the pan, off the heat, then add the flour, piri-piri seasoning, garlic and oil and toss to combine.

3 Tip the chips onto a foil-lined baking tray and spread out in an even layer. It is important that the chips are not on top of each other as they will not crisp in the oven if they are.

TO COOK

Transfer the chips to an oven preheated to 200°C/400°F/gas mark 6 for 30 minutes, until crisp and golden. Serve hot.

TO FREEZE

Set the par-boiled chips aside to cool to room temperature. Once cooled, cover the baking tray and transfer to the freezer for 2 hours to allow the chips to firm up. Transfer the part-frozen chips to a large, labelled freezer bag and freeze flat for up to 3 months.

TO COOK FROM FROZEN

The chips can be cooked directly from frozen. Tip the chips onto a foil-lined baking tray and spread out in an even layer, then transfer to an oven preheated to 200°C/400°F/gas mark 6 for 40 minutes, until crisp, golden and piping hot all of the way through.

LIGHTER CREAMED SPINACH

PREP: 5 MINS **COOK:** 10 MINS **SERVES:** 4 **SUGAR:** 6.8G **KCAL:** 127

I've never been a fan of spinach, but throw a bit of cream and garlic at it and I can't get enough! Unfortunately, traditional creamed spinach, though delicious, is best kept as a special-occasion treat. The good news is that I've lightened the recipe so you can still enjoy it as part of your healthy batching.

2 tsp low-fat margarine
½ cup (60g) frozen chopped onion
1 tsp garlic purée
2 tbsp plain flour
1½ cups (360ml) skimmed milk
½ tsp ground nutmeg
125g low-fat herb cheese (I use Boursin light)
450g fresh spinach, washed
salt and freshly ground pepper

1 Put the margarine in a large pan and place over a medium heat, until melted. Add the onions and garlic to the pan and cook, stirring continuously, for around 4 minutes, until soft.

2 Add the flour and stir through the onions for 30 seconds, to make a paste. Pour in the milk and stir again to combine. Leave to cook until the milk is warmed, but not boiling.

3 Add the nutmeg and herb cheese and whisk the mixture until the cheese has melted and the sauce is thick, smooth and lump-free.

4 Add the spinach to the pan and stir through the sauce. Cook, stirring occasionally, for 2 minutes, until the spinach has wilted. Remove from the heat and season to taste.

TO SERVE	TO FREEZE	TO REHEAT FROM FROZEN
The creamed spinach is now ready to serve.	Set the creamed spinach aside until cooled to room temperature, then transfer to a large, labelled freezer bag and freeze flat for up to 3 months.	Remove the creamed spinach from the freezer and leave to defrost fully in the fridge, ideally overnight. Once defrosted, tip the spinach into a baking dish, cover with foil and transfer to an oven preheated to 180°C/350°F/gas mark 4 for 15–20 minutes, until piping hot all of the way through.

SLICED CARROTS WITH GARLIC & TARRAGON

PREP: 3 MINS **COOK:** 10 MINS **SERVES:** 4 **SUGAR:** 6.4G **KCAL:** 50

This dish is a slightly unusual one for me as it needs to be made fresh, rather than for the freezer. It does use frozen carrots though, so can be on the table quickly and with minimum fuss. A great vegetable side dish for when you're running low on inspiration, but want something a bit more exciting than boiled veg to serve with your meal.

2½ cups (350g) pre-sliced frozen carrots
2 tsp low-fat margarine
2 tsp frozen chopped garlic
1 tsp dried or frozen chopped dill
1 tsp dried or frozen chopped tarragon
salt and freshly ground pepper

1 Add the carrots to a large pan and pour over boiling water to cover. Place over a medium heat and leave to cook for 5 minutes, until almost tender. Drain through a colander.
2 Return the pan to the heat and add the margarine. Once melted, add the garlic, dill and tarragon and stir to combine. Tip the carrots back into the pan and stir to coat in the herb 'butter'. Continue to cook, stirring occasionally, until the carrots are cooked to your liking.

TO SERVE

Season the carrots to taste, then serve hot. These are a wonderful accompaniment to steak, grilled chicken or fish.

LIGHT-AND-EASY NAAN BREADS

PREP: 15 MINS, PLUS RESTING **COOK:** 10 MINS **MAKES:** 6 NAANS **SUGAR:** 1.3G **KCAL:** 126

These naan breads are incredibly easy to make and they taste like the real deal! This recipe makes 6 small naans, but why not double-up and have a batch in the freezer for whenever you need them to mop up a curry?

1½ cups (175g) self-raising flour, plus extra for dusting
½ tsp baking powder
¾ cup (165g) low-fat Greek yoghurt
low-calorie cooking spray

1 Sift the flour and baking powder into a large mixing bowl, then add the yoghurt. Using a wooden spoon, stir the mixture until it comes together to form a rough dough.
2 Lightly dust the kitchen counter with flour, then turn the dough out and knead it briefly with your hands until everything comes together.
3 Divide the mixture into 6 equal-sized balls (around 60g each) and set aside somewhere warm for 30 minutes.

> If you are also making the Light-And-Easy Paprika Flatbreads, do so now while the naan dough is resting.

4 After 30 minutes, dust the kitchen counter again, then working with 1 ball of dough at a time, use a rolling pin to roll out each naan to a thickness of 2.5cm (1in). Repeat with the remaining balls of dough.
5 Spray a frying pan with low-calorie cooking spray and place over a medium heat. Once hot, add the naans in batches and cook for 2–3 minutes on each side until they are golden brown and tender all of the way through.

TO SERVE

The naan breads are now ready to serve. They make a wonderful accompaniment to any of the curries in this book.

TO FREEZE

Set the naan breads aside to cool to room temperature, then transfer to a large, labelled freezer bag and freeze flat for up to 3 months.

TO REHEAT FROM FROZEN

These can be defrosted before reheating or reheated straight from frozen. If defrosted, reheat in an oven preheated to 180°C/350°F/gas mark 4 for 8–10 minutes, until warmed through. If reheating from frozen, increase the reheating time to 10–12 minutes.

LIGHT-AND-EASY PAPRIKA FLATBREADS

PREP: 15 MINS **COOK:** 10 MINS **MAKES:** 6 FLATBREADS **SUGAR:** 2.5G **KCAL:** 122

These delicious flatbreads pair wonderfully with any of the Middle Eastern-inspired recipes from this book, or can be quickly dressed up with hummus and salad for a light and simple lunch.

1½ cups (175g) self-raising flour, plus extra for dusting
½ tsp baking powder
1 tsp smoked paprika
¾ cup (165g) low-fat Greek yoghurt
low-calorie cooking spray

1 Sift the flour, baking powder and smoked paprika into a large mixing bowl, then add the yoghurt. Using a wooden spoon, stir the mixture until it comes together to form a rough dough.

2 Lightly dust the kitchen counter with flour, then turn the dough out and knead it briefly with your hands until everything comes together.

3 Divide the mixture into 6 equal-sized balls (around 60g each), then working with 1 ball of dough at a time, use a rolling pin to roll out each flatbread to a thickness of 2.5cm (1in). Repeat with the remaining balls of dough.

4 Spray a frying pan with low-calorie cooking spray and place over a medium heat. Once hot, add the flatbreads in batches and cook for 2–3 minutes on each side until they are golden brown and tender all the way through.

TO SERVE

The flatbreads are now ready to serve. They are wonderful with kofta and hummus or served alongside the Turkey Tagine on p.178.

TO FREEZE

Set the flatbreads aside to cool to room temperature, then transfer to a large, labelled freezer bag and freeze flat for up to 3 months.

TO REHEAT FROM FROZEN

These can be defrosted before reheating or reheated straight from frozen. If defrosted, reheat in an oven preheated to 180°C/350°F/gas mark 4 for 8–10 minutes, until warmed through. If reheating from frozen, increase the reheating time to 10–12 minutes.

HARISSA DRESSING (OR DIP)

PREP: 3 MINS **SERVES:** 4
SUGAR: 3.8G **KCAL:** 55

I almost didn't put this recipe in the book because it's so embarrassingly simple, but it's a recipe that I come back to time and again as it is wonderful at turning an everyday meal into something that feels special. It can be made as a loose dressing by using yoghurt or a firmer dip by using quark cheese, so just pick the consistency that you want when it comes to making it. This isn't freezer-friendly, but takes so little time to make that prepping it for the freezer would be more complicated than making it from scratch.

1 cup (220g) low-fat Greek yoghurt or fat-free quark cheese
2 tsp harissa paste
fresh pomegranate seeds, to serve

1   Put the yoghurt or quark in a bowl, add the harissa paste and stir to combine, then scatter with the fresh pomegranate seeds.

TO SERVE

The dressing is now ready to serve. It is delicious drizzled over grilled meats or served with crudités for dipping. It will keep in a sealed jar in the fridge for 1 week.

LOW-FAT BLUE CHEESE DRESSING (OR DIP)

PREP: 3 MINS **SERVES:** 4
SUGAR: 2G **KCAL:** 70

This is another super-simple recipe that can be used as either a dressing when made with yoghurt, or a dip when made with quark. If, like me, you love the taste of blue cheese, then this is a great way to get more veg into your diet. I make a jar of it at the start of the week and enjoy it as a healthy snack throughout the week when served with raw vegetable batons.

1 cup (220g) low-fat Greek yoghurt or fat-free quark cheese
40g blue cheese, crumbled

1   Put the yoghurt or quark in a bowl, add the blue cheese and stir to combine.

TO SERVE

The dressing or dip is now ready to serve. It will keep in the a sealed jar in the fridge for up to 1 week.

LOW-FAT CAESAR DRESSING

PREP: 5 MINS **SERVES:** 4
SUGAR: 3.2G **KCAL:** 148

Caesar salad is delicious but can be packed with calories. Here's a brilliant low-fat version of the dressing to make in advance and keep in the fridge.

2 tbsp olive oil
1 cup (220g) low-fat Greek yoghurt
juice of 2 lemons
2 tbsp Dijon mustard
1 tsp garlic paste
2 anchovies, finely chopped
1 tsp Worcestershire sauce
⅓ cup (33g) pre-grated Parmesan cheese
salt and freshly ground pepper

1   Add all the ingredients to a freestanding blender and blend for around 15 seconds, until smooth.

The dressing is now ready to serve. It will keep in a sealed jar in the fridge for up to 1 week.

LOW-FAT RANCH SALAD DRESSING

PREP: 5 MINS **SERVES:** 4
SUGAR: 1.4G **KCAL:** 18

A great low-fat salad dressing that you can make in advance and keep in the fridge.

½ cup (110g) low-fat Greek yoghurt
1 tsp garlic puree
½ tsp onion salt
1½ tsp fresh lemon juice
1 small handful fresh chives, finely chopped
2 tbsp water

1   Put all the ingredients into a clean jam jar and seal the lid. Shake for 10–15 seconds, until everything is well combined.

The dressing is now ready to serve. It will keep in a sealed jar in the fridge for up to 1 week.

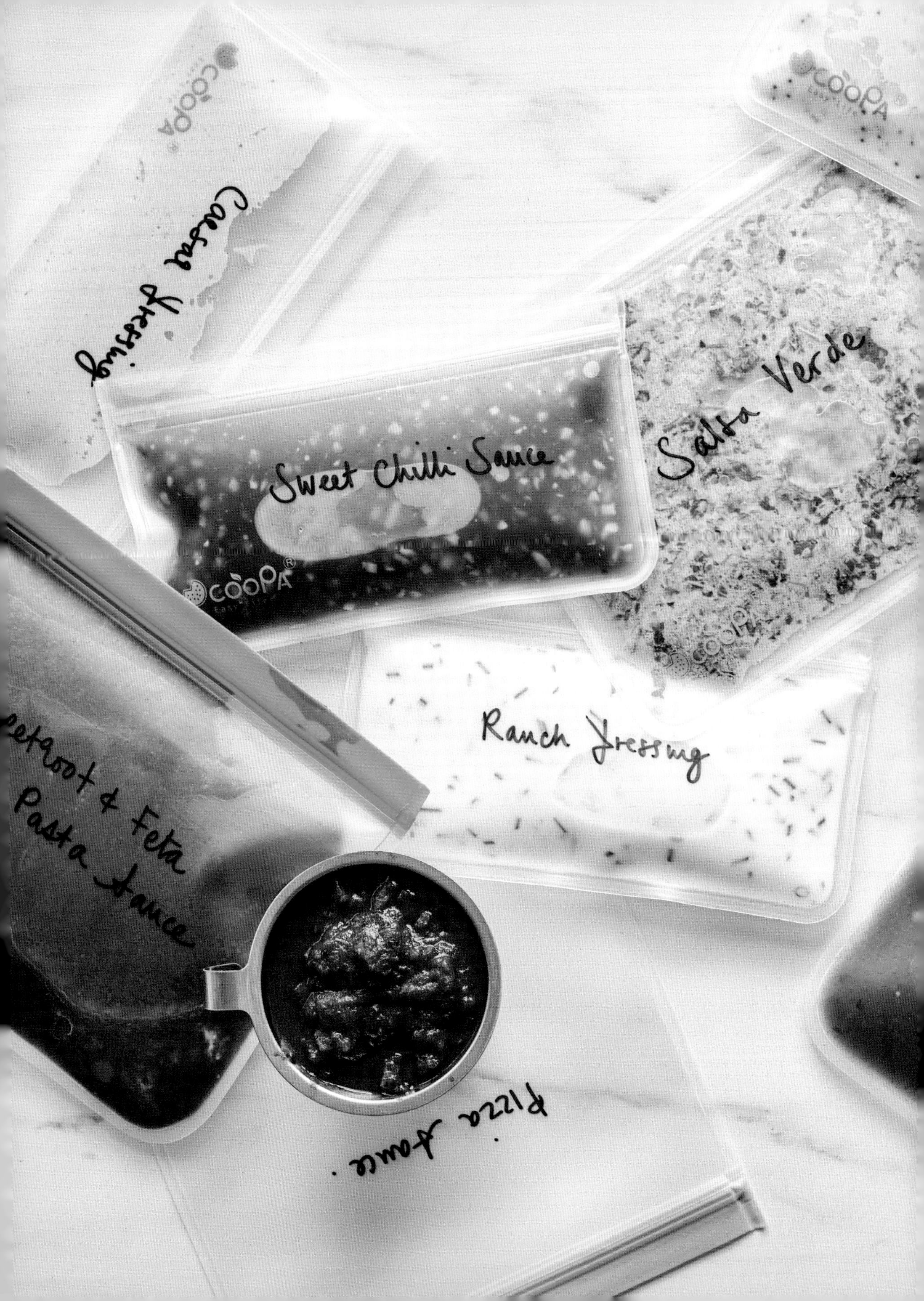

Caesar Dressing

Sweet Chilli Sauce

Salsa Verde

Ranch Dressing

Beetroot & Feta
Pasta Sauce

Pizza Sauce.

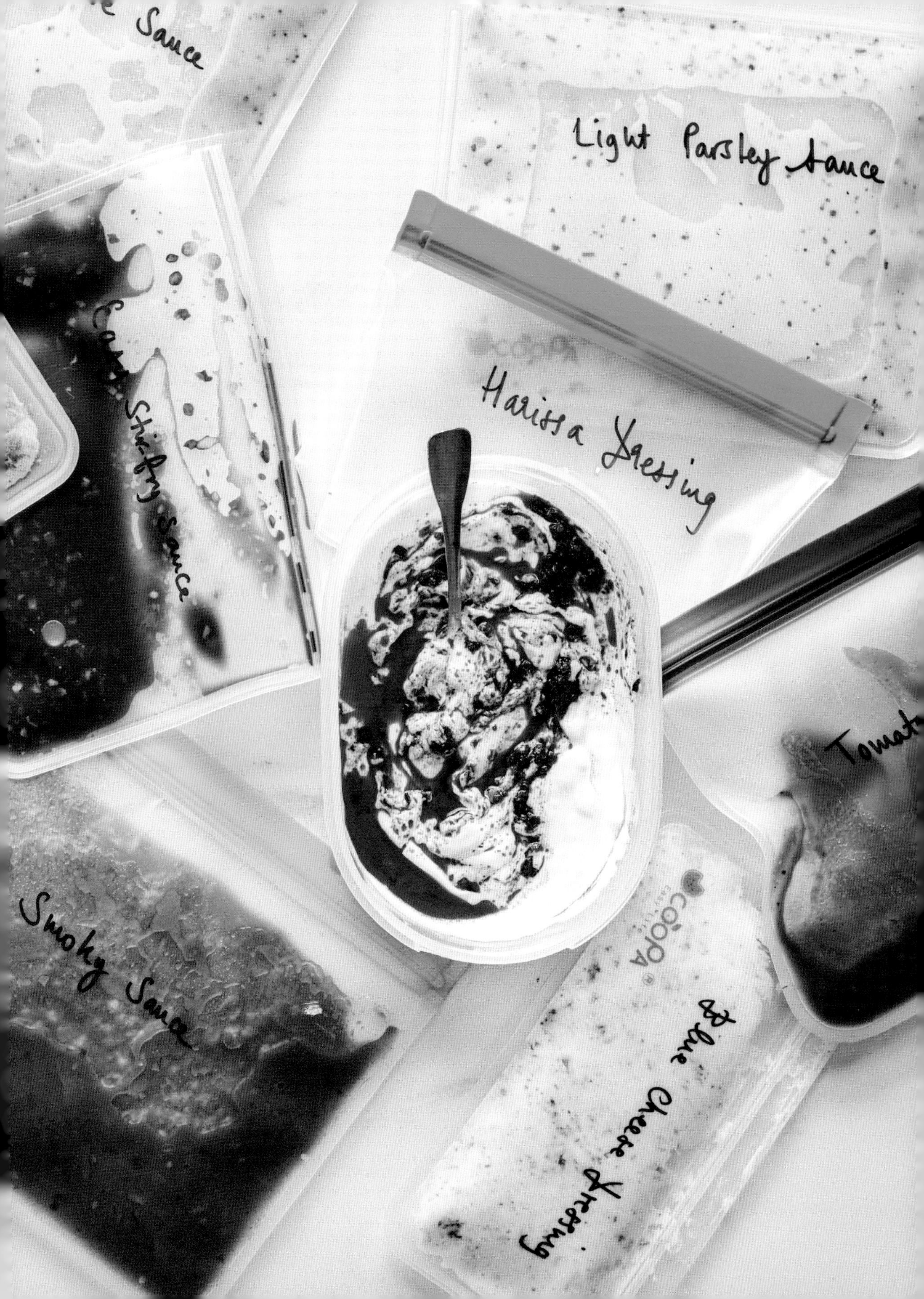

Sauce

Light Parsley Sauce

Egg Stuffing Sauce

Harissa Dressing

Smoky Sauce

Blue Cheese Dressing

Tomato

EASY STIR-FRY SAUCE

PREP: 5 MINS **SERVES:** 4 **SUGAR:** 3.4G **KCAL:** 63

This is a brilliant sauce to have on standby in the freezer as it is full of zing and can be added to stir-fries or used as a marinade for meat for an easy punch of flavour.

4 tbsp low-sodium soy sauce
1 tbsp homemade (p.215) or shop-
    bought sweet chilli sauce
1 tbsp sesame oil
1 tbsp cornflour
1 tsp frozen chopped ginger
1 tsp frozen chopped garlic

1 Put the soy sauce, sweet chilli sauce, sesame oil, cornflour, ginger and garlic into a small bowl and mix well to combine.

TO USE

The sauce is now ready to be used. It can be poured over meat as a marinade or added to stir-fries during cooking.

TO FREEZE

Transfer the sauce to a small, labelled freezer bag and freeze flat for up to 3 months.

TO USE FROM FROZEN

Remove the sauce from the freezer and leave it to defrost fully in the fridge. Once defrosted, use the sauce as described in the *To Use* section, left.

V

SWEET CHILLI SAUCE

PREP: 5 MINS **COOK:** 8 MINS **MAKES:** AROUND 1 CUP (240ML) **SUGAR:** 16G **KCAL:** 81

This is a wonderful sauce to make at home as you can control how much sugar goes into it, and the good news is that it's far easier than you might imagine. The sauce is sweet, but a little goes a long way and making it this way is healthier than using a shop-bought variety.

1 red chilli, deseeded and finely chopped
½ cup (120ml) white wine vinegar
½ cup (65g) brown sugar
1 tsp frozen chopped garlic
1 tsp hoisin sauce
1 tsp cornflour

1 Put the chilli, white wine vinegar, brown sugar, garlic and hoisin sauce in a small pan with ½ cup (120ml) of cold water. Place over a medium heat and bring to the boil, then reduce the heat to a gentle simmer and leave to cook for 5 minutes, stirring occasionally.
2 Meanwhile, put the cornflour in a small bowl, add 2 teaspoons of cold water and stir until smooth.
3 Add the cornflour mixture to the pan containing the rest of the ingredients and stir to combine. The sauce should thicken immediately. Continue to cook, stirring continuously to prevent the sauce from catching on the pan, for 2 minutes, then remove from the heat. Set aside to cool to room temperature.

TO USE

The sauce is now ready to use. It is wonderful served as a dip for Low-Fat Chicken Goujons (p.126), used to glaze salmon before cooking, or in a marinade or sauce for a stir-fry. It will keep in a sealed jar in the fridge for up to 2 weeks.

LIGHTER CHEESE SAUCE

PREP: 5 MINS **COOK:** 10 MINS **MAKES:** ABOUT 3 CUPS (720ML) **SUGAR:** 7.1G **KCAL:** 214

From cauliflower cheese to lasagne, so many of the best things are made with cheese sauce! This lighter version, made with skimmed milk and low-fat cheese, means that you don't have to skip these treats if you are watching what you eat.

1 tbsp low-fat margarine
3 tbsp plain flour
2½ cups (600ml) skimmed milk
1 cup (120g) low-fat, pre-grated
  cheddar cheese
1 tsp Dijon or wholegrain mustard
  (optional)
salt and freshly ground pepper

> If you are also making the Lighter Parsley Sauce, cook the two sauces side by side on the stove as the methods are very similar.

1 Heat the margarine in a large pan over a low-medium heat, until melted, then add the flour and cook, stirring, until the mixture has come together and thickened. Pour in a little of the milk and cook, whisking continuously, until the liquid has thickened. Keep adding more of the milk to the pan, whisking and thickening between each addition, until all of it has been used up and you have a thick, glossy white sauce.

2 Remove the pan from the heat and add the cheese and Dijon or wholegrain mustard, if using, then whisk until the cheese has melted into the sauce. Season to taste.

TO USE

The sauce is now ready to use. It can be used to dress pasta, spooned over cooked meat or fish or baked into a lasagne or macaroni cheese.

TO FREEZE

Set aside to cool to room temperature, then transfer to a large, labelled freezer bag (a zip-lock bag works best for this) and freeze flat for up to 3 months.

TO REHEAT FROM FROZEN

Remove the sauce from the freezer and leave to defrost fully in the fridge. Once defrosted, reheat in a pan until piping hot and use as described in the *To Use* section, left.

LIGHTER PARSLEY SAUCE

PREP: 5 MINS **COOK:** 10 MINS **MAKES:** ABOUT 3 CUPS (720ML) **SUGAR:** 7.2G **KCAL:** 179

This sauce pairs wonderfully with fish, whether spooned over grilled or baked fillets or baked into a fish pie. It freezes brilliantly, so I always have some of this on hand for a simple but delicious fish supper.

1 tbsp low-fat margarine
3 tbsp plain flour
2½ cups (600ml) skimmed milk
½ cup (50g) pre-grated Parmesan cheese
2 tsp frozen chopped parsley
salt and freshly ground pepper

1 Heat the margarine in a large pan over a low-medium heat, until melted, then add the flour and cook, stirring, until the mixture has come together and thickened. Pour in a little of the milk and cook, whisking continuously, until the liquid has thickened. Keep adding more of the milk to the pan, whisking and thickening between each addition, until all of it has been used up and you have a thick, glossy white sauce.

2 Remove the pan from the heat and add the Parmesan and parsley, then whisk until the cheese has melted into the sauce. Season to taste.

TO USE

The sauce is now ready to use. It can be used to dress fish, spooned over gammon or baked ham or baked into a fish pie.

TO FREEZE

Set aside to cool to room temperature, then transfer to a large, labelled freezer bag (a zip-lock bag works best for this) and freeze flat for up to 3 months.

TO REHEAT FROM FROZEN

Remove the sauce from the freezer and leave to defrost fully in the fridge. Once defrosted, reheat in a pan until piping hot and use as described in the *To Use* section, left.

TOMATO & CHILLI SAUCE

PREP: 5 MINS **COOK:** 20 MINS **MAKES:** ABOUT 3 CUPS (720ML) **SUGAR:** 12G **KCAL:** 112

1 tbsp olive oil
1 cup (115g) frozen chopped onions
1 tsp frozen chopped garlic
1 tbsp tomato purée
2 x 400g cans chopped tomatoes
½ tsp chilli flakes
1 tsp runny honey

1 Heat the oil in a large saucepan over a medium heat. Add the onions and garlic and cook, stirring continuously, for 2–3 minutes, until softened.
2 Add the tomato purée, chopped tomatoes, chilli flakes and honey to the pan and leave to cook, stirring occasionally, for 15–20 minutes, until reduced and thickened. If the sauce becomes too thick, add a splash of water to loosen. Remove from the heat.

TO USE

The sauce is now ready to use. It is great with meatballs or in a baked pasta dish, or could be used to dress wholewheat pasta for a simple lunch.

TO FREEZE

Set aside to cool to room temperature, then transfer the sauce to a large, labelled freezer bag and freeze flat for up to 3 months.

TO REHEAT FROM FROZEN

Remove the sauce from the freezer and leave to defrost fully in the fridge. Once defrosted, reheat in a pan until piping hot and use as described in the *To Use* section, left.

HOMEMADE PIZZA SAUCE

PREP: 5 MINS **COOK:** 20 MINS **MAKES:** ABOUT 3 CUPS (720ML) **SUGAR:** 11G **KCAL:** 71

2 x 400g cans chopped tomatoes
1 tbsp tomato purée
1 tsp dried basil
1 tsp runny honey

1 Put all of the ingredients in a large pan and place over a medium heat. Bring to the boil, then reduce the heat to a gentle simmer and cook, stirring occasionally, for 20 minutes, until thickened and reduced.

TO USE

The sauce is now ready to use. It is great for topping pizzas, but could also be used to dress pasta for a simple lunch.

TO FREEZE

Set the sauce aside to cool to room temperature. Transfer the mixture to a large, labelled freezer bag or, if you want to freeze in smaller portions, spoon into a plastic ice-cube tray. Freeze flat for up to 3 months.

TO USE FROM FROZEN

Remove the sauce from the freezer and leave to defrost fully in the fridge or, if you are in a hurry, defrost slowly in the microwave. If using on a pizza, the sauce does not need to be reheated once defrosted; simply dress the pizza and bake.

SMOKY SAUCE

PREP: 5 MINS **COOK:** 5-10 MINS **SERVES:** 4 **SUGAR:** 10G **KCAL:** 99

This is a great sauce to have in the freezer for dressing up simple grilled meats. It also makes a great accompaniment to the Chipotle Turkey Meatballs on page 147. The chipotle paste imparts a mellow smoky flavour with just a hint of spice, so feel free to ramp it up or down to suit your family's tastes.

1 tbsp olive oil
1 cup (115g) frozen chopped onions
1 tsp frozen chopped garlic
2 x 400g cans chopped tomatoes
½ tsp chipotle paste
½ cup (120ml) low-sodium
   vegetable stock
½ tsp runny honey or sugar
salt and freshly ground pepper

1   Place the olive oil in a saucepan over a medium heat, then add the onions and garlic and cook, stirring, for 2–3 minutes, until soft.
2   Add the chopped tomatoes, chipotle paste, vegetable stock and honey or sugar to the pan and stir to combine. Bring to the boil, then reduce the heat to a gentle simmer and leave to cook, stirring occasionally, for 20 minutes, until the sauce has reduced and thickened. Remove the pan from the heat and season to taste.

TO SERVE

The sauce is now ready to be served. It makes a great companion to grilled meats or is wonderful served over pasta.

TO FREEZE

Leave the sauce to cool to room temperature, then transfer to a large, labelled freezer bag and freeze flat for up to 3 months.

TO REHEAT FROM FROZEN

Remove the sauce from the freezer and allow to defrost fully in the fridge, ideally overnight. Once defrosted, heat the sauce in a large pan over a medium heat for 5–10 minutes, stirring occasionally, until piping hot all of the way through.

DESSERTS

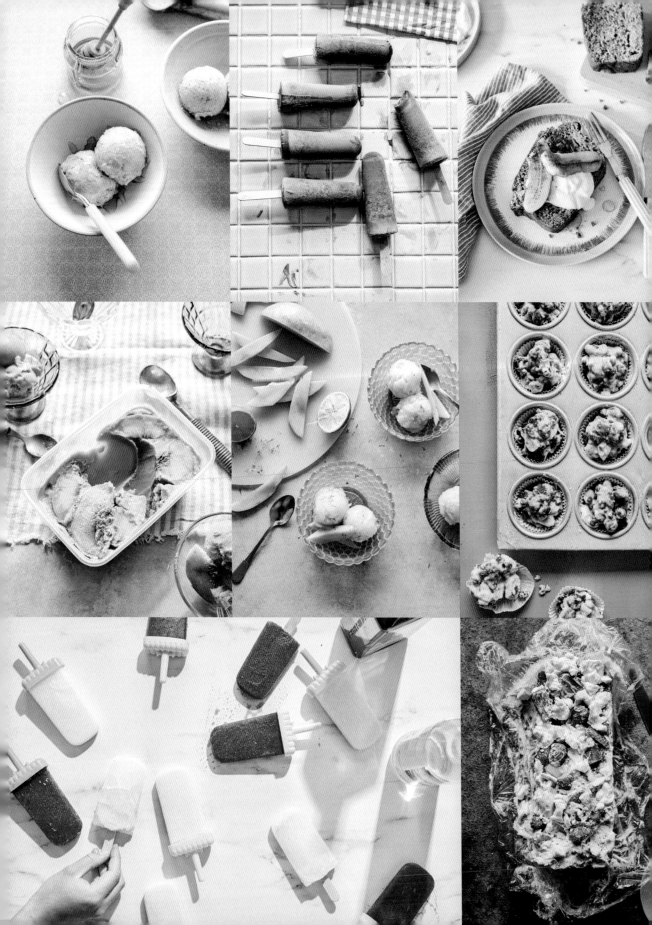

DESSERTS

Desserts are a special-occasion treat, but that doesn't mean that we should deny ourselves when we fancy something sweet. The recipes in this chapter are designed to satisfy your sweet tooth without causing feelings of regret afterwards.

You'll notice that I have a lot of recipes for frozen treats here, this is because when I fancy something sweet I often want it immediately, so waiting for something to defrost or cook from frozen isn't really an option! Ice lollies and sorbets can be eaten straight from the freezer, are a great alternative to ice cream and can be packed with delicious, naturally sweet fruit for a sweet, but relatively healthy, treat.

For sit-down meals and dinner parties, you can't go wrong with my recipes for Lighter Chocolate & Raspberry Pots (p.230), Jam-Jar Blueberry & Lemon Cheesecakes (p.246) or Semifreddo Eton Mess (p.247), all of which feel special and celebratory. And for the times when you want a slice of cake to enjoy in the afternoon with a cup of tea, my Lighter Banana Bread (p.242) can be made ahead, stored in the freezer and defrosted in individual slices, so you needn't have the temptation of a whole cake sitting on the kitchen counter. Enjoy!

GIN & TONIC ICE LOLLIES

PREP: 5 MINS, PLUS 4 HRS CHILLING **MAKES:** 6 **SUGAR:** 2.4G **KCAL:** 37

These lollies are the perfect adult summer treat to enjoy in the sun. For this recipe, and those that follow on the next couple of pages, you will need a 6-hole lolly mould. The good news is that these can be picked up cheaply and, once you have used them a couple of times, you will have more than recouped the spend in money saved buying shop-bought lollies.

6 lemon slices, halved
70ml gin
1 cup (240ml) slimline tonic water
1 tbsp agave nectar

1   Add 2 half-slices of lemon to each of your lolly moulds.
2   Add the gin, tonic water and agave nectar to a small jug and stir to combine.
3   Pour the gin-and-tonic mixture into the lolly moulds and push in the lolly sticks.

TO FREEZE

Transfer the filled lolly moulds to the freezer and freeze for at least 4 hours, but ideally overnight. These will keep in the freezer for up to 3 months.

TO SERVE FROM FROZEN

Remove the lollies from the freezer to serve as needed.

RASPBERRY LEMONADE
ICE LOLLIES

PREP: 5 MINS, PLUS 4 HRS CHILLING **MAKES:** 6 **SUGAR:** 1.6G **KCAL:** 20

I wanted to pair the grown-up lollies (opposite) with something that the whole family could enjoy, and this recipe definitely fits the bill. Both sweet and tart, these mouth-puckering lollies are the perfect antidote to the wilting heat of a long summer day.

2 cups (480ml) diet lemonade
1 cup (135g) frozen raspberries
juice of 1 lemon

1   Pour the lemonade into a large jug and stir until most of the bubbles have disappeared.
2   Pour the lemonade into a freestanding blender along with the frozen raspberries and lemon juice. Blend until smooth.
3   Pour the raspberry-lemonade mixture into the lolly moulds and push in the lolly sticks.

TO FREEZE

Transfer the filled lolly moulds to the freezer and freeze for at least 4 hours, but ideally overnight. These will keep in the freezer for up to 3 months.

TO SERVE FROM FROZEN

Remove the lollies from the freezer to serve as needed.

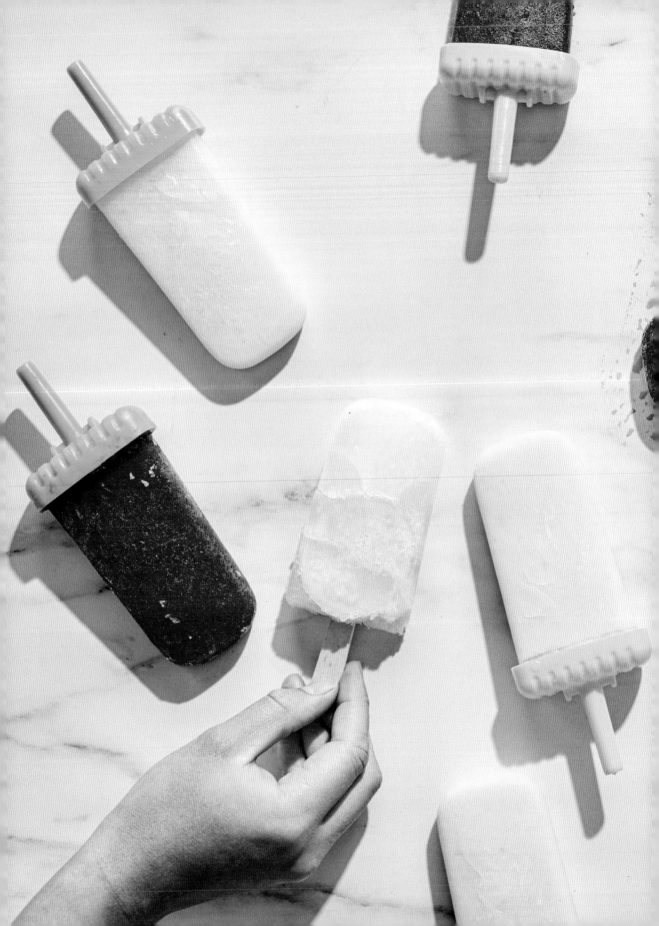

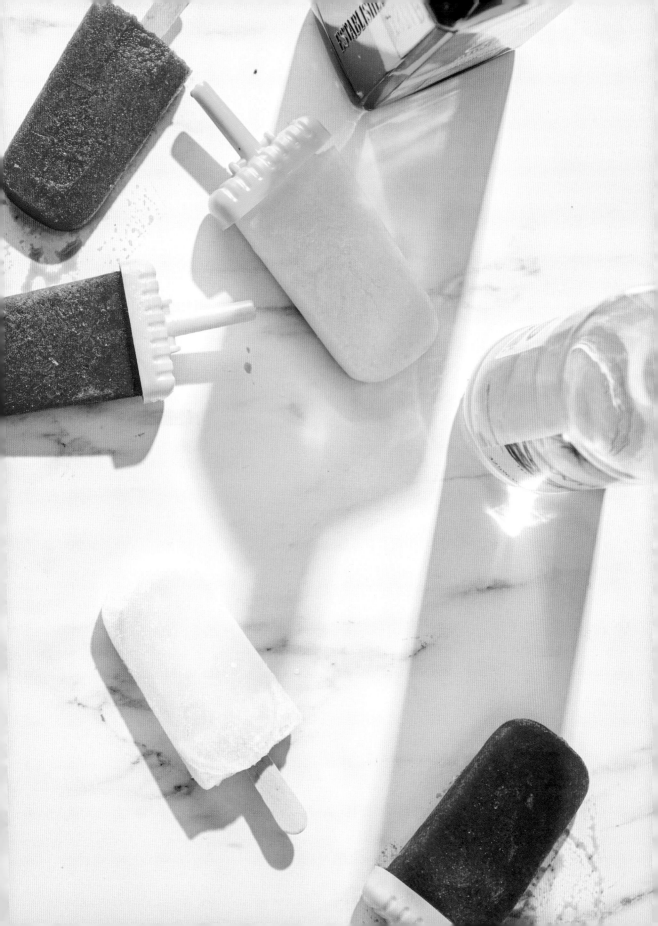

PINA COLADA ICE LOLLIES

PREP: 10 MINS, PLUS 4 HRS CHILLING **MAKES:** 6 **SUGAR:** 11G **KCAL:** 121

These boozy lollies will transport you straight to a tropical beach. If you want to make a kid-friendly version, simply omit the booze when making the lollies.

1 cup (170g) canned pineapple chunks in juice
½ cup (120ml) juice from canned pineapple (above)
2 tbsp white rum
2 tbsp agave nectar
1 cup (240ml) reduced-fat coconut milk

1   Add all of the ingredients to a freestanding blender and blend until smooth.
2   Pour the pina-colada mixture into the lolly moulds and push in the lolly sticks.

TO FREEZE

Transfer the filled lolly moulds to the freezer and freeze for at least 4 hours, but ideally overnight. These will keep in the freezer for up to 3 months.

TO SERVE FROM FROZEN

Remove the lollies from the freezer to serve as needed.

RASPBERRY DAIQUIRI ICE LOLLIES

PREP: 5 MINS, PLUS 4 HRS CHILLING **MAKES:** 6 **SUGAR:** 6.5G **KCAL:** 33

Another boozy lolly to bring the party on a hot summer's day. These work just as well with or without the rum, so remove it for a more family-friendly version, or why not make both? Do make sure that the boozy versions are clearly labelled as 'adults only' in the freezer!

1 cup (120g) frozen raspberries
juice of 1 lime
1 cup (240ml) water
2 tbsp white rum
2 tbsp runny honey or agave
 nectar

1 Add all of the ingredients to a freestanding blender and blend until smooth.
2 Pour the raspberry-daiquiri mixture into the lolly moulds and push in the lolly sticks.

TO FREEZE

Transfer the filled lolly moulds to the freezer and freeze for at least 4 hours, but ideally overnight. These will keep in the freezer for up to 3 months.

TO SERVE FROM FROZEN

Remove the lollies from the freezer to serve as needed.

LIGHTER CHOCOLATE & RASPBERRY POTS

PREP: 10 MINS, PLUS 4–5 HRS CHILLING **SERVES:** 4 **SUGAR:** 22G **KCAL:** 359

These dark and decadent chocolate pots are free from refined sugars and heavy cream, making them lighter than the usual variety. The milk can be substituted for a plant-based alternative if you prefer and you can use whatever berries you have to hand. These make a great do-ahead dinner-party dessert, as you can simply whip them out of the freezer when you are serving the main course and they will be perfectly defrosted and ready to serve come dessert time.

2 handfuls fresh raspberries
200g dark chocolate
¾ cup (180ml) semi-skimmed milk
1 egg, beaten
2 tbsp maple syrup

1 Divide the raspberries between the bases of 4 ramekin dishes and set aside.
2 Break the chocolate into a heatproof mixing bowl and set aside.
3 Put the milk in a small saucepan and heat over a low heat until just starting to simmer, then pour it over the chocolate. Leave to sit for 1 minute to allow the chocolate to melt, then whisk the chocolate and milk to a smooth paste.
4 Add the beaten egg and maple syrup to the chocolate mixture and whisk again to combine.
5 Pour the chocolate mixture into the ramekins over the top of the raspberries, dividing the mixture evenly between each ramekin.

TO SERVE
Transfer the ramekins to the fridge and leave to set for 4–5 hours, until just firm but not solid. The chocolate pots are now ready to serve.

TO FREEZE
Cover and label the ramekins and freeze for up to 3 months.

TO SERVE FROM FROZEN
Remove the ramekins from the freezer and set aside at room temperature to defrost for 30–40 minutes, until still firm but not solid. The chocolate pots are now ready to serve.

CHOCOLATE MINI MILKS

PREP: 10 MINS, PLUS 4 HRS CHILLING **MAKES:** 6 **SUGAR:** 15G **KCAL:** 93

A lighter version of everyone's favourite childhood ice lolly. Feel free to mix up the flavour on these and sub the chocolate for puréed strawberry or banana instead. Whatever flavour you choose, they won't last long in the freezer.

½ cup (120ml) light condensed milk
1 tbsp cocoa powder
1½ cups (360ml) semi-skimmed milk

1 Add the condensed milk and cocoa powder to a mixing bowl and whisk until well combined and there are no lumps of cocoa in the mixture. Add the milk and whisk again to combine.
2 Pour the chocolate milk mixture into the lolly moulds and push in the lolly sticks.

TO FREEZE

Transfer the filled lolly moulds to the freezer and freeze for at least 4 hours, but ideally overnight. These will keep in the freezer for up to 3 months.

TO SERVE FROM FROZEN

Remove the lollies from the freezer to serve as needed.

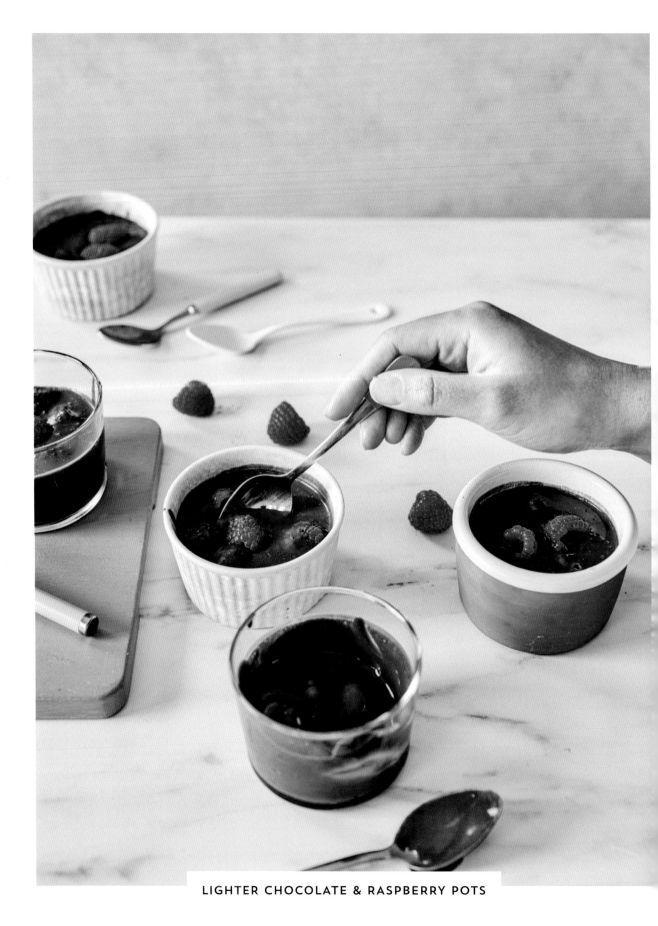

LIGHTER CHOCOLATE & RASPBERRY POTS

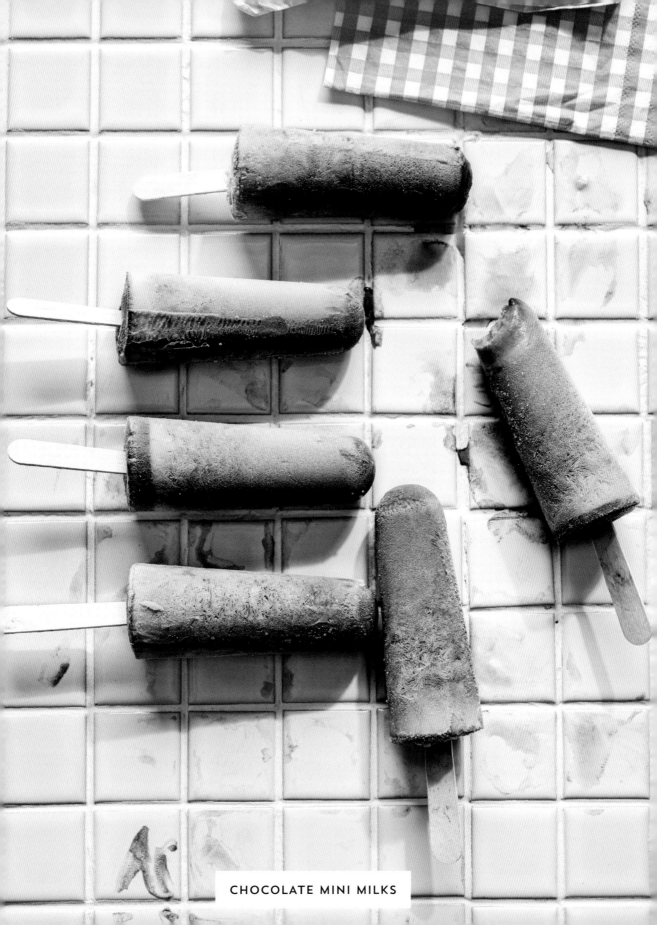

CHOCOLATE MINI MILKS

FROZEN YOGHURT & BERRY CUPCAKE BITES

PREP: 5 MINS, PLUS CHILLING **MAKES:** 12 **SUGAR:** 9.9G **KCAL:** 149

These frozen cupcake bites are a wonderfully healthy frozen snack to have in the freezer for whenever you need to satisfy your sweet tooth. They are always a hit with the kids in my house, so are a great way to avoid the call of the ice-cream van and get some fruit in!

12 tbsp granola
½ cup (60g) frozen raspberries
½ cup (65g) frozen blueberries
1 banana, finely chopped
2 tbsp honey
1½ cups (330g) Greek yoghurt

1   Line a 12-hole muffin tin with muffin cases, then add a tablespoon of granola to the base of each case.
2   Add the raspberries, blueberries, chopped banana, honey and yoghurt to a large bowl and stir to combine, then divide the mixture between the muffin cases, spooning over the top of the granola.

TO FREEZE

Transfer the muffin tin to the freezer until the yoghurt mixture is firm, then transfer the cupcake bites to a large, labelled freezer bag in a single layer and freeze flat for up to 3 months.

TO SERVE FROM FROZEN

These are served from frozen, so simply grab one from the freezer whenever you need a healthy, sweet treat.

STRAWBERRY & PEACH FROZEN YOGHURT

PREP: 5 MINS, PLUS 4 HRS CHILLING **SERVES:** 4 **SUGAR:** 20G **KCAL:** 160

Frozen yoghurt is a much lighter alternative to ice cream and has the added benefit of being far easier to make! It freezes much firmer than ice cream, so do let it soften out of the freezer for 15 minutes or so before scooping.

1 cup (150g) frozen strawberries
1 cup (150g) frozen peach slices
  or 2 fresh ripe peaches, peeled,
  pitted and chopped
2 cups (220g) Greek yoghurt
3 tbsp runny honey

1 Place all of the ingredients in a food processor and process until smooth and combined.

TO FREEZE

Pour the mixture into a labelled tub with a lid, then cover and freeze for up to 3 months.

TO SERVE FROM FROZEN

Remove from the freezer and set aside to soften for around 15 minutes, until scoopable. Then use an ice-cream scoop or spoon to scoop into bowls and serve.

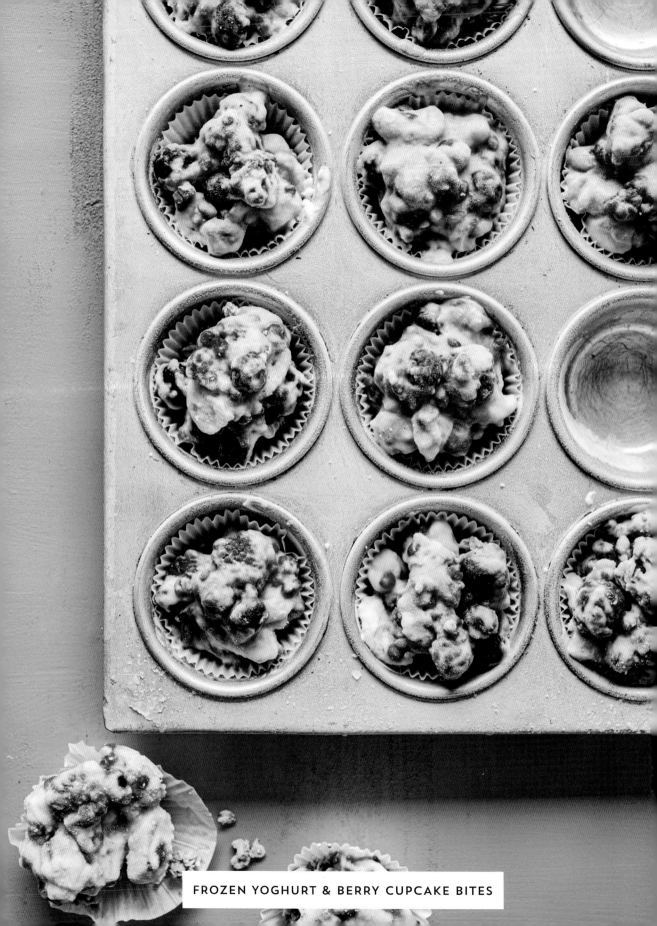

FROZEN YOGHURT & BERRY CUPCAKE BITES

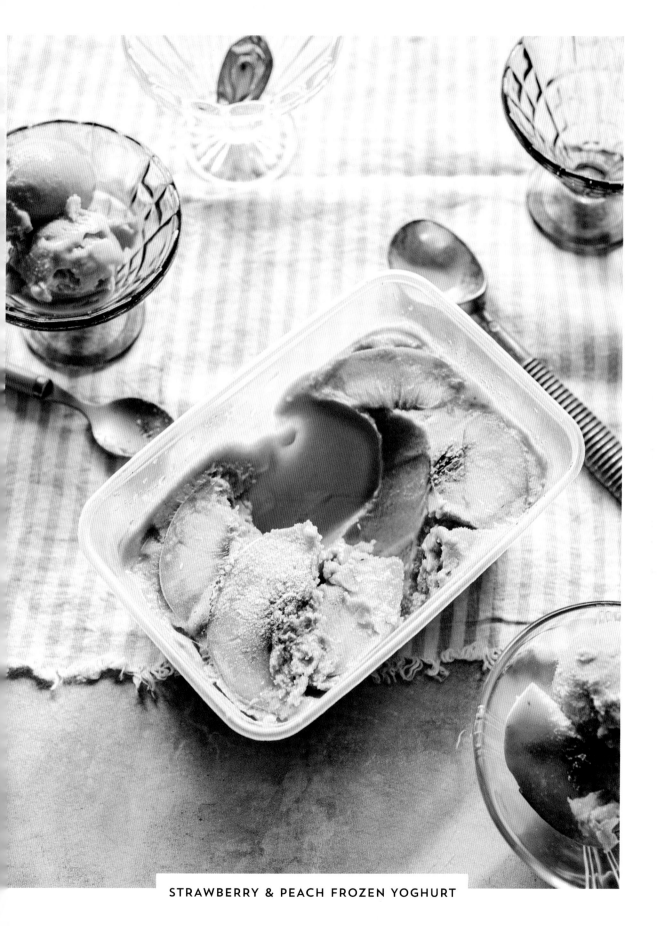

STRAWBERRY & PEACH FROZEN YOGHURT

MANGO & LIME SORBET

PREP: 10 MINS, PLUS 4 HRS CHILLING **SERVES:** 4 **SUGAR:** 47G **KCAL:** 198

This bright and zesty sorbet makes a great, lighter alternative to ice cream and is wonderful served as it is or with fresh fruit on the side.

2 large mangoes, peeled, pitted
and flesh roughly chopped
1 cup (125g) icing sugar
zest and juice of 2 limes

1 Place all of the ingredients in a food processor and process until smooth and combined.

TO FREEZE

Pour the mixture into a labelled tub with a lid, then cover and freeze for 1 hour. Remove the sorbet from the freezer and stir to break up any ice crystals, then return to the freezer for another 3 hours, when it will be firm and ready to eat. The sorbet will keep in the freezer for up to 3 months.

TO SERVE FROM FROZEN

Remove from the freezer and set aside to soften for around 15 minutes, until scoopable. Then use an ice-cream scoop or spoon to scoop into bowls and serve.

RASPBERRY & STRAWBERRY SORBET

PREP: 10 MINS, PLUS 4 HRS CHILLING SERVES: 4 SUGAR: 40G KCAL: 190

This is made with frozen berries, so providing you have a well-stocked freezer, can easily be knocked up with without the need for a special trip to the shops. Feel free to play with the flavours and use whatever berries you have to hand.

2 cups (240g) frozen raspberries
2 cups (300g) frozen strawberries
juice of 1 lemon
1 cup (125g) icing sugar
½ cup (120ml) water

1 Place all of the ingredients in a food processor and process until smooth and combined.

TO FREEZE

Pour the mixture into a labelled tub with a lid, then cover and freeze for 1 hour. Remove the sorbet from the freezer and stir to break up any ice crystals, then return to the freezer for another 3 hours, when it will be firm and ready to eat. The sorbet will keep in the freezer for up to 3 months.

TO SERVE FROM FROZEN

Remove from the freezer and set aside to soften for around 15 minutes, until scoopable. Then use an ice-cream scoop or spoon to scoop into bowls and serve.

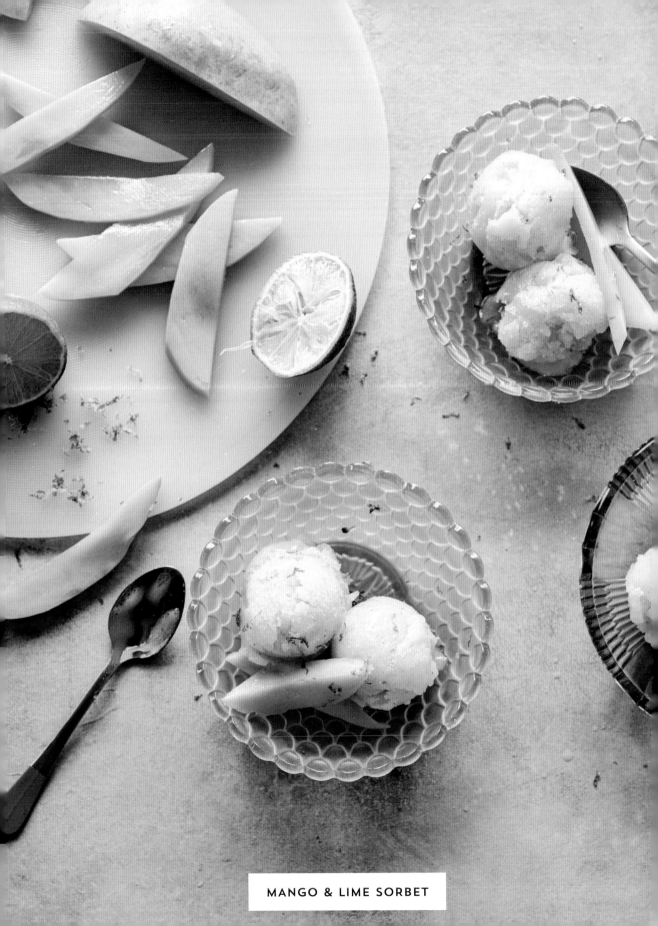

MANGO & LIME SORBET

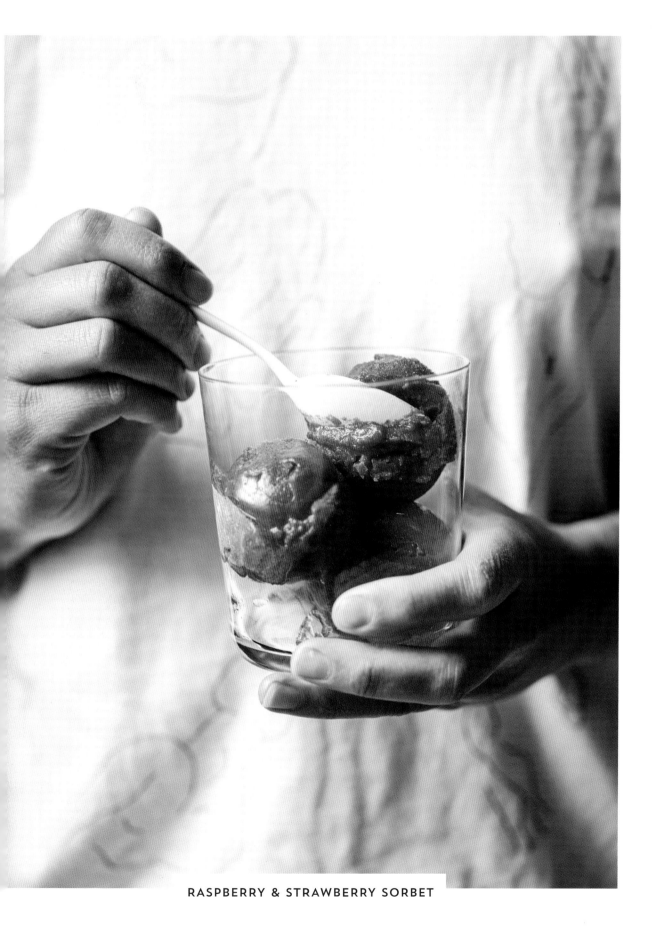

RASPBERRY & STRAWBERRY SORBET

LIGHTER BANANA BREAD

PREP: 10 MINS **COOK:** 1 HR 10 MINS **MAKES:** 1 X 900G (2LB) LOAF CAKE
SUGAR: 18G **KCAL:** 264

This is a lighter version of the banana bread recipe that you can find in my meal planner book. Here, maple syrup takes the place of refined sugar and wholemeal flour is used instead of white, to make something that still feels like a treat but is that little bit kinder to the waistline.

⅓ cup (75g) low-fat margarine
½ cup (145g) maple syrup
2 eggs, beaten
½ cup (110g) low-fat Greek yoghurt
1¾ cups (210g) wholemeal flour
1 tsp bicarbonate of soda
1 tsp vanilla extract
3 ripe bananas

1 Preheat the oven to 160°C/300°F/gas mark 3. Grease a 900g (2lb) loaf tin with margarine and line with greaseproof paper.
2 In a microwave or small pan, melt the margarine, then pour into a large mixing bowl with the maple syrup and beaten eggs and stir to combine.
3 Add the yoghurt, flour, bicarbonate of soda and vanilla extract to the bowl and mix until just combined.
4 In a separate small bowl, mash the bananas with a fork, then add to the rest of the ingredients and gently fold into the mixture with a wooden spoon.
5 Pour the mixture into the prepared loaf tin and level out with a spoon.
6 Transfer to the oven and bake for 1 hour–1 hour 10 minutes until golden, well risen and an inserted skewer comes out clean. Set aside to cool in the tin.

TO SERVE

Once cooled, turn the cake out of the tin, cut into slices and serve.

TO FREEZE

Once cooled, turn the cake out of the tin, cut into slices and wrap each in a layer of clingfilm followed by a layer of foil. Freeze the slices flat. Store in the freezer for up to 3 months.

TO SERVE FROM FROZEN

Remove individual slices of the cake from the freezer as needed and set on the counter to defrost. They should be ready to eat in around 30 minutes.

BANANA & HONEY FROZEN YOGHURT

PREP: 5 MINS, PLUS 4 HRS CHILLING **SERVES:** 4 **SUGAR:** 36G **KCAL:** 255

Frozen banana adds a creaminess to this frozen yoghurt that transforms into something much more akin to ice cream, but with none of the bad stuff!

4 ripe bananas
1 x 450g tub honey-flavoured
  Greek yoghurt
2 tbsp runny honey, plus extra for
  decoration

1   Place all of the ingredients in a food processor and process until smooth and combined.

TO FREEZE

Pour the mixture into a labelled tub with a lid, then drizzle a little extra honey over the top as a decoration. Cover and freeze for 4 hours, after which time it will be ready to serve. The frozen yoghurt will keep in the freezer for up to 3 months.

TO SERVE FROM FROZEN

Remove from the freezer and set aside to soften for around 15 minutes, until scoopable. Then use an ice-cream scoop or spoon to scoop into bowls and serve.

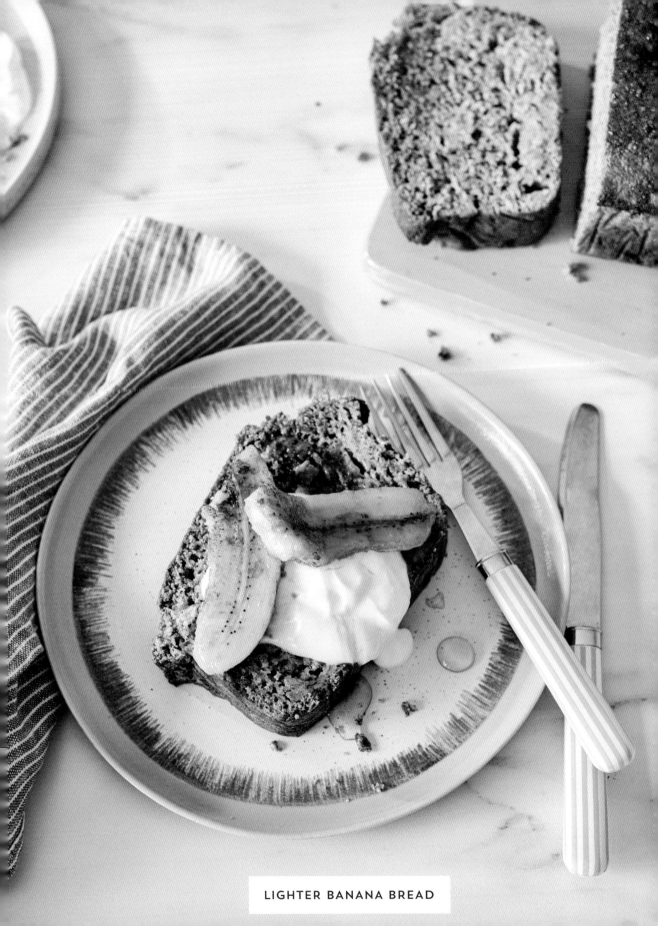

LIGHTER BANANA BREAD

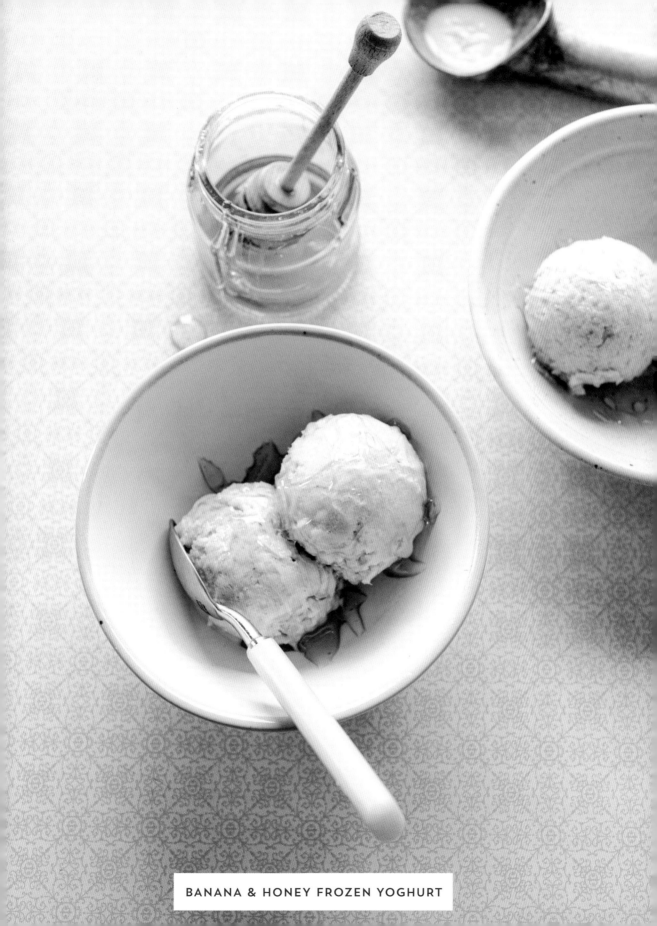

BANANA & HONEY FROZEN YOGHURT

JAM JAR BLUEBERRY & LEMON CHEESECAKES

PREP: 10 MINS, PLUS 2HRS CHILLING **SERVES:** 4 **SUGAR:** 72G **KCAL:** 577

These are a great low-fat alternative to a traditional cheesecake that the whole family will love! Serving these in little jars not only makes them look sweet, but also helps with portion control. They can be made ahead and defrosted as needed, so are a perfect dessert for low-fuss entertaining.

¼ cup (50g) low-fat margarine

8 reduced-fat digestive biscuits, crushed

scant ½ cup (100ml) semi-skimmed milk

1 x 36g pack Bird's no-added-sugar Dream Topping

scant 1 cup (180g) low-fat cream cheese.

zest and juice of 1 lemon

½ cup (75g) fresh blueberries, plus a few extra to decorate

1 Add the margarine to saucepan and place over a low heat until melted. Remove from the heat and tip the crushed digestive biscuits into the pan. Stir to combine.

2 Divide the 'buttered' biscuit mixture between 4 small jars or ramekins and press down firmly to form a base. Set aside.

3 Add the milk and powdered Dream Topping to a mixing bowl and whisk with a handheld electric whisk until starting to thicken.

4 Add the cream cheese and lemon zest and juice and whisk again until smooth.

5 Fold the blueberries through the mixture, then spoon over the biscuit bases, dividing the cheesecake mixture evenly between the jars or ramekins.

6 Scatter a extra few blueberries over the top of each cheesecake for decoration.

TO SERVE

Transfer the cheesecakes to the fridge for 2 hours to set. The mixture should be firm and creamy, but not solid. The cheesecakes are now ready to serve.

TO FREEZE

Cover and label the jars or ramekins and freeze for up to 3 months.

TO SERVE FROM FROZEN

Remove the cheesecakes from the freezer and leave to defrost fully in the fridge, ideally overnight. The cheesecakes are now ready to serve.

SEMIFREDDO ETON MESS

PREP: 5 MINS, PLUS 6-8 HRS CHILLING **SERVES:** 6 **SUGAR:** 54G **KCAL:** 300

This is my lighter take on everyone's favourite summer dessert. It contains all of the delicious elements of the original, but is served as a semifreddo and is much lighter on the cream! This is a wonderful thing to have in your freezer, as you can remove slices as and when you need them and return the rest to the freezer for another day.

1 x 405g can light condensed milk
1 cup (220g) low-fat Greek
  yoghurt
½ cup (120ml) single cream
1 cup (150g) fresh strawberries,
  hulled and finely chopped
1 cup (150g) fresh blueberries
4 shop-bought meringue nests,
  crushed

1 Line a 900g (2lb) loaf tin with clingfilm, leaving some excess overhanging the sides of the tin. Set aside.
2 Add the condensed milk, yoghurt and single cream to a mixing bowl and stir until well combined. Add the fruit and meringue pieces to the bowl and fold through the mixture.
3 Pour the mixture into the prepared loaf tin and level out. Bring up the sides of the clingfilm to cover the top of the mixture.

TO FREEZE

Transfer the semifreddo to the freezer and freeze for 6–8 hours, until set. The semifreddo is now ready to serve, but will keep in the freezer for up to 3 months.

TO SERVE FROM FROZEN

Remove the semifreddo from the freezer and set aside for 5 minutes to defrost slightly. Using the clingfilm, lift the semifreddo from its tin and place on a chopping board. Slice as many slices as needed from the semifreddo, transfer to serving plates and serve. Any remaining semifreddo can be put back in the tin, re-covered and returned to the freezer until needed.

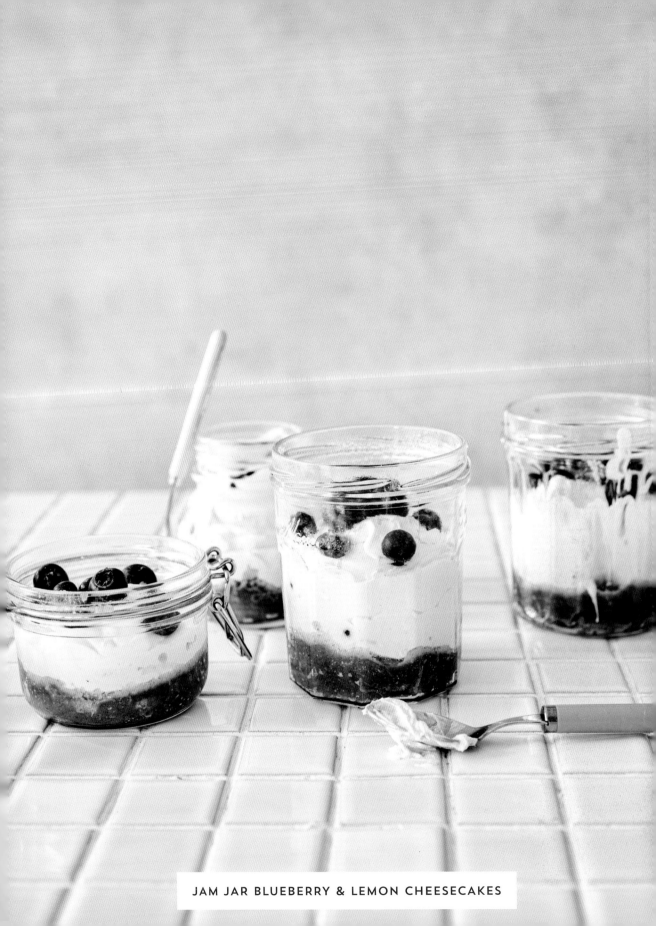

JAM JAR BLUEBERRY & LEMON CHEESECAKES

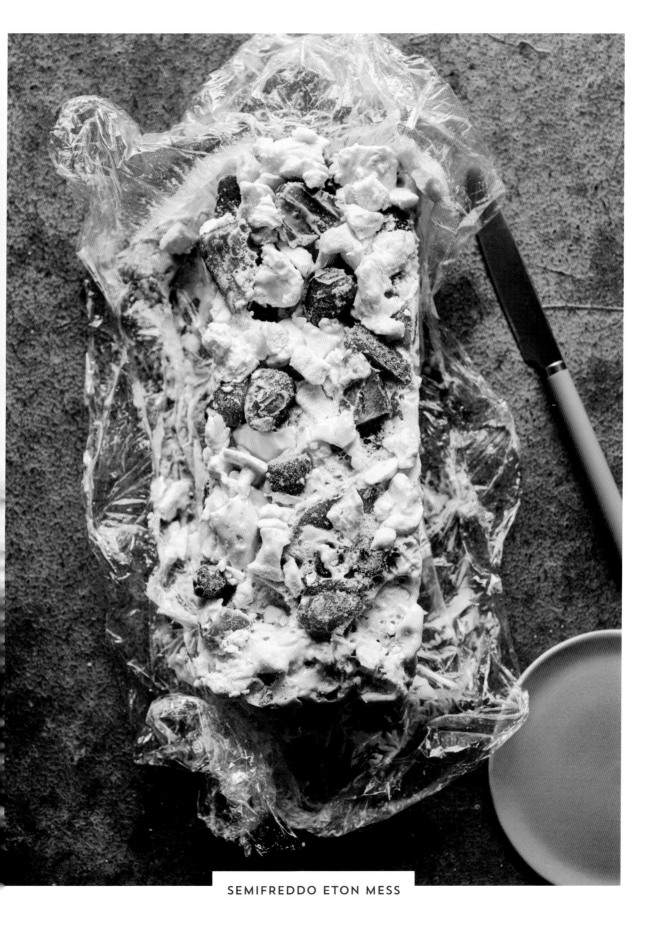

SEMIFREDDO ETON MESS

INDEX

ACKNOWLEDGEMENTS

Well, another book is complete and, as always, there's no way I could have done it without all the people in my life who have helped guide and support me through the many stages of bringing it into the world. To everyone who follows me on social media, has taken the time to like or comment on my posts, has visited my website, has tried my recipes or has spread the word in any way – you are all part of The Batch Lady. We are a team and without you it simply couldn't happen. Every day I am thankful to have you all along with me on this journey.

To all of my wonderful friends (you know who you are), I thank you for sticking with me as I forge along with the mad Batch-Lady world that I have created, and for all your support when things sometimes go in unexpected directions! It is very liberating to know that you can do something completely different in your 40s and that your friends will be your loudest cheerleaders. For that I will be forever grateful.

A huge thanks to Cathryn Summerhayes, my agent at Curtis Brown, who is, as always, a wealth of information and reassures and gives me great guidance in all the projects I undertake.

To the 'batch-it crew' at HQ, Harper Collins, who continue to 'believe in the batch!'. Lisa Milton, Kate Fox, Nira Begum and the rest of the team, your belief has allowed these books to become a reality. I shall be forever grateful for the experience and can only hope to write many more books with such an amazing and professional team.

To Dan Hurst, my wonderful project editor. I'm at the stage where I don't think I would ever like to write a book without you. As always, you have made this book look and sound amazing. It always astounds me how you take my hundreds of word documents and spreadsheets and make them come alive in a book. And to Georgina Hewitt, my designer, who always amazes me with the way she can take my most complex recipes, such as the *3 for the Fridge, 3 for the Freezer* sections in this book, and not only squeeze them onto a page designed for a single recipe, but also make them look beautiful! Thank you, both.

Liz Haarala and Max Hamilton, thank you for the fab photographs. We have had to overcome so many hurdles in 2020, but a highlight is definitely being able to get the last photographs done in Scotland, just days before we all locked down again. A brilliant job done. Also, a huge thank you to the food-stylist team, Sam Dixon, Rosie French and Rosie Ramsden, who made my dishes look so beautiful.

A massive shout out has to go to Nicola Bruce, who is now firmly part of The Batch Lady crew. You worked tirelessly in helping to perfect these recipes, through times when lockdown and Covid-19 saw us struggling to get supplies, but seeing your smiling face on Zoom was always a bonus.

Of course, a massive thank you goes to my lovely husband, Peter, who is my rock. Thank you for putting up with me and for holding the fort every time I disappeared to write, and for finally agreeing to have your photo in the book!

Last, but certainly not least, thank you to my two children, Jake and Zara. You were brilliant at keeping busy over their summer holidays as I worked to finish the first draft of this book in time. You are both amazing and so supportive – thank you for being proud of what your mummy does and for being amazing at what you do!